THE TOXIC SCHOOLHOUSE

Edited by

Madeleine Kangsen Scammell
Boston University School of Public Health

Charles Levenstein
University of Massachusetts Lowell

Work, Health, and Environment Series
***Series Editors*: Charles Levenstein, Robert Forrant, and John Wooding**

Routledge
Taylor & Francis Group
NEW YORK AND LONDON

First published 2014 by Baywood Publishing Company, Inc.

Published 2017 by Routledge
605 Third Avenue, New York, NY 10017
4 Park Square, Milton Park, Abingdon, Oxon OX14 4RN

First issued in hardback 2017

Routledge is an imprint of the Taylor & Francis Group, an informa business

ISBN 13: 978-0-89503-851-7 (pbk)
ISBN 13: 978-0-41578-567-9 (hbk)

Library of Congress Cataloging-in-Publication Data

The toxic schoolhouse / edited by Madeleine Kangsen Scammell, Charles Levenstein ; series editors, Charles Levenstein, Robert Forrant, and John Wooding.
p. ; cm. -- (Work, health, and environment series)
Includes bibliographical references and index.
ISBN 978-0-89503-851-7 (paper) -- ISBN 978-0-89503-852-4 (e-pub) -- ISBN 978-0-89503-853-1 (e-pdf)
I. Scammell, Madeleine Kangsen, editor of compilation. II. Levenstein, Charles, editor of compilation. III. Series : Work, health, and environment series.
[DNLM : 1. Environmental Exposure--prevention & control--Canada. 2. Environmental Exposure--prevention & control--United States. 3. Schools–Canada. 4. Schools--United States. 5. Environmental Health--Canada. 6. Environmental Health--United States. 7. Environmental Pollutants--Canada. 8. Environmental Pollutants--United States. 9. Safety Management--Canada. 10. Safety Management--United States. WA 799]
HQ770.7
363.11'9371--dc23

2013027281

We dedicate this book to

Malala Yousafzai

for her work to ensure that education is a basic human right.

Table of Contents

Preface

In the Baywood series *Work, Health, and Environment,* the conjunction of topics is deliberate and critical. We begin at the point of production—even in the volumes that address environmental issues—because that is where things get made, workers labor, and raw materials are fashioned into products. It is also where things get stored or moved, analyzed or processed, computerized or tracked. In addition, it is where the folks who do the work are exposed to a growing litany of harmful things or are placed in harm's way. The focus on the point of production provides a framework for understanding the contradictions of the modern political economy.

Despite claims to a post-industrial society, work remains essential to all our lives. While work brings income and meaning, it also brings danger and threats to health. The point of production, where goods and services are produced, is also the source of environmental contamination and pollution. Thus, work, health, and environment are intimately linked.

Work organizations, systems of management, indeed the idea of the "market" itself, have a profound impact on the handling of hazardous materials and processes. The existence or absence of decent and safe work is a key determinant of the health of the individual and the community: what we make goes into the world, sometimes improving it, but too often threatening the environment and the lives of people across the globe.

We began this series to bring together some of the best thinking and research from academics, activists, and professionals, all of whom understand the intersection between work and health and environmental degradation, and all of whom think something should be done to improve the situation.

The works in this series stress the political and social struggles surrounding the fight for safer work and protection of the environment, and the local and global struggle for a sustainable world. The books document the horrors of cotton dust, the appalling and dangerous conditions in the oil industry, the unsafe ways in which toys and sneakers are produced, the struggles to link unions and communities to fight corporate pollution, and the dangers posed by the petrochemical industry, both here and abroad. The books speak directly about the contradictory effects of the point of production for the health of workers, community, and the environment. In all these works, the authors keep the politics front and foremost. What has emerged, as this series has grown, is a body of scholarship uniquely focused and highly integrated around themes and problems absolutely critical to our own and our children's future.

Acknowledgments

We wish to thank Jennifer Ames for her hard work, determination, and good humor while putting this book together. It can truly be said that this book would not have happened without her. We would also like to acknowledge the support and inspiration of the Massachusetts Teachers Association's (MTA's) Environmental Health and Safety Committee; and of Phil Katz and Michael Sireci, field representatives of the MTA. Sarah Gibson, Grace Sembajwe, and Chris Oliver made intellectual contributions that are beyond measure and not adequately reflected in the pages within. We are grateful for their work to protect environmental health. Craig Slatin, editor extraordinaire of *New Solutions: A Journal of Environmental and Occupational Health Policy*, provided editorial advice and guidance for our special issue, and Nancy Irwin Maxwell was an excellent editor. Fred Sperounis provided advice and insight, good humor and delightful company over Japanese luncheons.

Of course, nothing could have been published were it not for the writers. Thank you for your contributions. We also thank Ellen Loeb and Muna Kangsen for their support.

Introduction

Schools were once central to the life of every community in the United States, and children, at least in popular rhetoric and federal legislation, are not to be left "behind." According to the U.S. Environmental Protection Agency (EPA), more than 53 million children and about 6 million adults spend a substantial part of their days in elementary and secondary schools [1]. The National Institute for Occupational Safety and Health (NIOSH) describes the "education sector" as the second-largest industry in the United States with 13,155,000 workers (including "Primary and Secondary Schools, Technical and other Colleges, Universities, Professional Schools, Educational Support" in its calculations) [2]. In Massachusetts alone during the academic year 2008-2009, more than 72,000 teachers were employed in public schools, in settings ranging from early childhood education through high school [3]. Yet, despite their large numbers, teachers and other school staff are often working under environmental conditions that are, to say the least, problematic.

Even in Massachusetts, considered by many to be an unusually progressive and innovative state for education, ranking in the top of the country by a variety of performance measures [4, 5], we have serious environmental threats to the health of workers and students. Between 2003 and 2006, the Massachusetts Department of Environmental protection (MassDEP) conducted inspections of 56 public schools uncovering a number of violations of state and federal laws including [6]:

- lead/copper levels in water from bubblers/sinks higher than the state action level, which is 15 parts per billion for lead and 1.3 parts per million for copper;
- improper storage and handling of hazardous chemicals and hazardous waste;
- unnecessary idling of buses for more than 5 minutes; and
- failures to update Asbestos Management Plans or to keep them on site, and to notify MassDEP of asbestos removal or demolition work.

In 2006, the Massachusetts Department of Public Health (MassDPH) reported problems in the state's public schools involving heating, ventilation, and air-conditioning operations; indoor microbial growth; and indoor and outdoor sources of respiratory irritants, vapors, gases, and particulates. Further, 13 percent of work-related asthma cases reported to MDPH were among those who worked in educational services [6]. Other state departments were focusing on similar inspections.

On top of these concerns, reports of PCB contamination of schools in the Commonwealth became more frequent. Pittsfield, Massachusetts, was already notorious because of PCB contamination by General Electric, including the gifts of PCB-contaminated topsoil to schools and parks in the town. New Bedford was also reported to have PCB contamination, not only in its harbor but also in brownfield sites near schools. Construction workers found PCBs when renovating buildings at the University of Massachusetts Amherst, and an investigation of Boston schools by Harvard researchers determined that there was widespread PCB contamination. When the Massachusetts Teachers Association's Environmental Health and Safety Committee began discussion of the PCB issue, professionals in occupational safety and health warned the committee not to adopt the U.S. EPA approach to asbestos in the schools because "AHERA does not work."

The claim that AHERA (the Asbestos Hazard Emergency Response Act) does not work, and would not be a good model for regulation of school hazards, has some justification. Although federal legislation for managing asbestos problems in public schools has existed since the late 1980s, there has been no peer-reviewed evaluation of the efficacy of such legislation since 1991. Through our own research we obtained annual summary reports submitted by the Massachusetts Division of Occupational Safety (MassDOS) to EPA Region I for the years 1998-2008. The reports identify for each year the number of compliance audits that MassDOS conducted, the identity of the schools whose AHERA programs MassDOS audited, whether MassDOS issued a Notice of Non-Compliance (NNC) or the equivalent, and the number of violations included in each NNC. For the period for which we obtained annual summary reports, MassDOS audited an average of 30.7 schools per year. On average, 88 percent of MassDOS's audits resulted in the issuance of an NNC. The average number of violations per NNC was 8.7, and compliance did not improve over time.

Much of the "policy" work in occupational and environmental health and safety has involved passing legislation and/or the establishment of standards and regulations for government and its agencies to implement or enforce. We have neglected the implementation aspects of policy, however, perhaps because we have fallen prey to the myth that passing the law solves the problem. We move on to the next problem, assuming that the policies are our solutions. Consequently, we have neglected the tricky fields of implementation—including management, inspection, audit, the creation of effective incentives, and punishment. In many cases the success of our policies is reliant on an engaged and forceful citizenry that is not afraid of getting the runaround, dogged in its determination, and with all the time in the world to find what should be in plain sight. Many of the case studies in this book are stories that rely on advocates in systems that are meant to be dependent on citizen-based enforcement. Is this a solution? We don't think so.

We are concerned by the inadequate attention paid to school environments and important issues concerning the siting and construction of schools, indoor air quality, the safety of school drinking water, the efficacy of restrictions on pesticide use, and the problem of toxic cleaners. No systematic approach for addressing these school-based hazards exists.

Increasing public interest in brownfields, waste sites, and environmental justice has highlighted school issues as they pertain to children's environmental health, but the occupational health issues of school staff have been neglected. While teachers are more likely than workers in many other service or manufacturing industries to be union members, the physical and social hazards they face in the workplace do not rank high on the public social agenda. Teachers and their organizations have been important actors in school policy—including school environmental health—but not without challenges by conservative political forces. The recent struggle in Chicago is an example of tensions between teachers and their employers.

The politics and economics of the education environment, we believe, have not been thoroughly discussed in the occupational and environmental health policy literature despite being raised by activists and advocates (e.g., the Center for Health, Environment and Justice). Our hope with this book is to at least raise these issues from a variety of perspectives.

This work was originally conceived as a special issue of *New Solutions: A Journal of Environmental and Occupational Health Policy* [7], and we have used most of that collection of articles as chapters—updated by their authors—in this book. We have supplemented those articles with additional chapters that we think help to fill out the picture.

The chapters are presented in three groupings: First, we have a selection of articles that describe the problems of school health and environment. The chapter by Paulson and Barnett of the Healthy Schools Network discusses the problem of coordination and responsibility for the school environment, raising a question for which we have no answer: "Who's in Charge?" This is followed by a report by Tolle Graham and Jean Zotter on the health effects of deteriorating conditions in the Boston schools. Yanna Lambrinidou, Simoni Triantafyllidou, and Marc Edwards then present a report on the failure of the school systems across the nation to address the problem of lead in drinking water. This is an old problem (like asbestos), and it is shocking that the hazard persists. Robert Herrick's paper on PCBs follows; again, it is disturbing that this well-known hazard has not been addressed fully. Finally, Cohen presents the problem of school siting, an issue that underscores the economics that underpins the school environment problem. Communities pressed for funds by the national attack on public spending—and by the local conservative backlash against taxes—find their way to brownfields and swamps to save money on school construction. Cohen's article addresses the policy framework and authorities regarding school siting and construction.

The second section of the book features chapters on struggles to defend the school environment. We were anxious to include the voices of activists, so the first two chapters of this section report on interviews with teachers and school activists from the United States and Canada. In the third chapter of this section, Eileen Senn discusses the close relationship between New Jersey's state affiliate of the National Education Association and the Work Environment Council, and their successful efforts to promote a union-led defense of school environments. Gibson and Levenstein report on a Massachusetts case in which union, parents, and school officials negotiated clean air conditions. And Laura Senier et al. then discuss the coalition of custodians and parents who have been fighting for the use of less toxic cleaners in schools.

In the final section of the book we present three chapters on relatively progressive policies to address school environment problems. Taylor et al. argue for federal attention to the use of pesticides in school environment. Parker reviews the various legal reforms to contain the explosion of asthma in children. And finally, Ames and Levenstein discuss the Massachusetts School Building Authority as an approach to more comprehensive control of the school environment.

Of course, this collection of writing is not definitive in any sense. We have not addressed the issue of hydraulic fracturing on school property, for example [8], a very important environmental health issue in the news as we go to press. This book suggests one more arena in which it is important to have discussion and debate among environmentalists, trade unionists, health and safety advocates, community (and parent) activists, and the public health scientific community.

NOTES

1. U.S. Environmental Protection Agency, *Healthy Schools: Lessons for a Clean Educational Environment*, http://www.epa.gov/region1/children/pdfs/healthy_schools.pdf (accessed September 26, 2012).
2. National Institute for Occupational Safety and Health, "NIOSH Program Portfolio," http://www.cdc.gov/niosh/programs/pps/sector.html (accessed February 22, 2012).
3. A. Owens, Harvard Kennedy School, *The Massachusetts Teacher Workforce: Status and Challenges*, http://www.hks.harvard.edu/var/ezp_site/storage/fckeditor/file/pdfs/centers-programs/centers/rappaport/paes/owens_teachers.pdf (accessed February 22, 2012).
4. National Assessment of Educational Progress, "The Nation's Report Card," http://nationsreportcard.gov/ (accessed September 26, 2012).
5. P. E Peterson, L. Woessmann, E. A. Hanushek, & C. X. Lastra-Anadon, Harvard's Program on Education Policy and Governance & Education Next, Taubman Center for State and Local Government, Harvard Kennedy School, *Globally Challenged: Are U.S. Students Ready to Compete?*, http://www.hks.harvard.edu/pepg/PDF/Papers/PEPG11-03_GloballyChallenged.pdf (accessed September 26, 2012).
6. A. Ranger (ed.), Massachusetts School Building Authority, *Environmental Health and Safety Problems Reported In Massachusetts' Public Schools, By Massachusetts Agencies* [unpublished report], updated February 2006. Available from the editor at: aranger@msba.state.ma.us, 617-720-4466.

7. M. K. Scammell and C. Levenstein (eds.), School Health and Environment, special issue of *New Solutions: A Journal of Environmental and Occupational Health Policy* 20(1).
8. D. Boucher, "Natural Gas Wells Proposed on Capital High Grounds," *Charlestown Daily Mail*, October 8, 2012, http://dailymail.com/News/201210070158 (accessed October 8, 2012).

Madeleine Kangsen Scammell
Charles Levenstein
Boston, Massachusetts, October 10, 2012

PART I

The Problem

CHAPTER 1

Who's in Charge of Children's Environmental Health at School?

Jerome Paulson and Claire Barnett

Children spend many hours each week in and around school buildings. Their short- and long-term health outcomes and ability to learn are affected by numerous environmental factors related to the school buildings, the school grounds, the school transportation system, and the use of various products and materials in and around the school. Many school buildings are old; these schools, and even newer buildings, can contain multiple environmental health hazards. While some districts report that they have environmental health policies in place, no independent verification of these policies or their quality exists. Teachers and other staff, but not children—who are more vulnerable to hazards than adults—are afforded some protections from hazards by Occupational Safety and Health Administration (OSHA) regulations, by their employment contracts, or through adult occupational health services. Major environmental problems include: indoor air quality, lighting, pests and pesticides, heavy metals and chemical management issues, renovation of occupied buildings, noise, and cleaning processes and products. No agency at the federal or state levels is charged with ensuring children's health and safety in and around school buildings. No systematic means exists for collecting data about exposures that occur in the school setting. Recommendations are made for dealing with issues of data collection, federal actions, and state and local actions, and for building the capacity of the Pediatric Environmental Health Specialty Units (PEHSUs) designated and funded by the Environmental Protection Agency and the Centers for Disease Control and Prevention in responding to and evaluating risks to children's environmental health in schools.

Just as adult health is impacted by exposures and injuries in the workplace, the environments in which children spend time can influence their health. Children spend many hours each week in and around school buildings, and their short- and long-term health outcomes, as well as their learning, are affected by numerous environmental factors related to the school buildings, the school grounds, the school transportation system, and the use of various materials in and around the school. Teachers' health and productivity may also be affected.

It is widely recognized that children are generally more vulnerable to environmental health hazards than adults [1-3]. For example, children breathe more air and drink more water per unit of body mass than adults do. Therefore, if the air or water that they are consuming is polluted, they receive a larger dose of that pollution. Children also have a longer "shelf life" than adults. If time from exposure to manifestation of toxicity is 40 years, a child is more likely to live long enough to develop the toxicity. Children are more likely to be closer to the ground or on the ground than adults. For example, their exposure to pesticides that have precipitated or been sprayed at ground level will be greater than an adult's exposure. Infants in child care centers are not able to move themselves out of harm's way. For example, young children have a limited capacity to protect themselves from exposure to the sun to avoid sunburn. Toddlers are much more likely to put objects in their mouths than older children or adults, again increasing their risk of exposure. While children are school-aged—from preschool to grade 12—cells in the body are migrating, metabolic pathways are forming, and hormonal systems are changing. All of these differences between children and adults, singularly and cumulatively, make children's responses to environmental toxicants different from those of adults.

The following issues need to be addressed regarding children's environmental health issues in American schools:

1. Numerous environmental health hazards are present in U.S. schools including, but not limited to, poor indoor air quality, hazards associated with lighting, pests and pesticides, noise, radon, asbestos, lead, polychlorinated biphenyls (PCBs), drinking water contamination, cleaning processes and products, and siting problems.
2. The protection of adults and children from these environmental health hazards:
   a. is inadequate for both children and adults, although adult employees of schools have a patchwork of regulatory and other protections; and
   b. is not designed to take into account the needs of children, who outnumber adults in schools, or, in many cases, those of pregnant teens and women.
3. The present system for gathering data about school-related environmental health problems is inadequate or nonexistent.
4. There are no baseline data on children's illnesses, injuries, and exposures in schools and on school facilities that include environmental conditions.

The nation must build a system for collecting and analyzing data relevant to children's environmental health, one that will protect and intervene for children at risk of harm. Improvements to adult environmental health protections are also required, although that is not the focus of this chapter.

REVIEW OF CURRENT STATUS

In the United States, about 132,000 public and private schools are operated by approximately 15,000 school districts and independent entities, and serve 55 million children [4]. About 70 percent of schools enroll elementary students; 24 percent, secondary students; and the remainder, both [5]. Schools are also the worksite for about 7 million adults serving as teachers, administrators, and support staff [4].

In the late 1990s, the average age of school buildings in the United States was 42 years; some of the buildings were over 100 years old [6]. Even the best facilities, which are well sited, designed, and constructed, need continuing maintenance and repair, but schools have deferred these items for years [1]. Any building may have a myriad of problems: poor indoor air quality, lighting, and noise control; routine use of highly toxic pesticides; presence of radon, asbestos, lead, or PCBs; inadequate heating, lighting, and plumbing systems; poor drinking water quality; unsafe playgrounds; or poor siting [7, 8].

The most detailed information about the status of American school buildings in the states is the Government Accounting Office's (GAO) study on "The Condition of American Schools" [5] which was undertaken in the mid-1990s and is based on self-reports that were not independently verified. There is no evidence to suggest that the environmental health status of the schools has improved markedly since that time. In fact, the National Center for Education Statistics (NCES) produced a report in 2000, also based on self-reports and not independently verified, which found similar needs and underscored the need for funding [9]. The GAO found (see Table 1) that "[a]bout 50 percent of the schools reported at least one unsatisfactory environmental condition; while 33 percent reported multiple unsatisfactory conditions. Of those, half reported four to six unsatisfactory conditions. Those conditions most frequently reported to be unsatisfactory were acoustics for noise control, ventilation, and physical security.

In addition, three-quarters of schools responding had "spent funds during the [early 1990s] on requirements to remove or correct hazardous substances such as asbestos (57 percent), lead in water or paint (25 percent), materials [in underground storage tanks] such as fuel oil (17 percent), radon (18 percent), or other requirements (9 percent)." The GAO found that an additional "two-thirds [of schools] must spend funds [between 1994 and 1997] to comply with these same requirements—asbestos (45 percent), lead (18 percent), [underground storage tanks] (12 percent), radon (12 percent), or other requirements

Table 1. Percent of Public Schools Rating the Condition of Building Features as Less than Adequate, by School Characteristics: 1999 [5]

School characteristic	At least one building feature is in less than adequate condition	Roofs	Framing, floors, foundations	Exterior walls, finishes, windows, doors	Interior finishes, trim	Plumbing	Heating, ventilation, air conditioning	Electric power	Electrical lighting	Life safety features
All public schools	50	22	14	24	17	25	29	22	17	20
School instructional level										
Elementary school	49	22	14	23	17	24	28	21	17	19
High school	56	26	16	27	20	28	34	25	19	22
Combined	54	18	15	31	14	25	34	20	20	29
School enrollment size										
Less than 300	55	24	19	31	20	28	29	23	19	26
300 to 599	50	22	12	21	16	27	32	21	17	21
600 or more	49	22	14	23	18	20	26	22	16	16

Locale										
Central city	56	23	12	27	20	28	30	26	18	21
Urban fringe/large town	44	19	13	21	16	21	27	21	15	17
Rural/small town	52	25	17	25	17	26	31	19	20	23
Region										
Northeast	39	16	10	18	14	19	22	14	10	11
Midwest	51	20	15	28	15	25	27	19	15	19
South	51	25	15	22	16	24	28	22	20	22
West	57	27	16	26	25	32	40	32	22	27
Percent minority enrollment										
5 percent or less	48	21	15	26	14	22	28	18	16	18
6 to 20 percent	49	25	15	23	17	26	29	18	16	22
21 to 50 percent	46	17	12	17	14	23	25	19	15	18
More than 50 percent	59	28	14	29	24	29	34	32	23	24
Percent of students in school eligible for free or reduced-price school lunch										
Less than 20 percent	45	18	14	21	17	23	28	18	14	16
20 to 39 percent	45	21	11	21	14	23	26	20	15	18
40 to 69 percent	53	22	16	25	14	23	29	21	18	22
70 percent or more	63	32	17	30	26	32	35	30	24	27

(8 percent) [1]." This amounted to about $2.3 billion to correct or remove hazardous substances, primarily asbestos, and a need to expend about $5 billion more to bring all schools up to the then-existing federal requirements [1]. The NCES survey found that three-fourths of schools needed to repair, renovate, or modernize buildings to put them into good condition, and that 43 percent of schools reported that at least one of the six environmental conditions was unsatisfactory [6]. Ventilation was most often reported (26%) as inadequate, and the estimate of repair costs was put at $127 billion [6].

While there is information on the total dollar volume of school construction nationwide, there is no reliable information on whether environmental issues are being systematically addressed and resolved. In the same study, the GAO found that "28 million [students] attend schools nationwide that need one or more building feature extensively repaired, overhauled, or replaced or that contain an environmentally unsatisfactory condition." (Environmental factors include lighting, heating, ventilation, indoor air quality, acoustics for noise control, energy efficiency, and physical security of buildings [1].)

Schools more recently self-reported on a CDC survey that they have policies in place to deal with many environmental health issues: about one-third of districts and one-half of schools report having an indoor air quality management program; about one-third report school bus engine idling reduction policies; 80-plus percent of school districts had policies related to hazardous materials; around 90 percent of schools reported plans for hazardous materials; and one-quarter of state education officials surveyed reported that they required districts to have an integrated pest management plan [10].

Issues that have not been systematically addressed encompass:

- infiltration of fumes and carbon monoxide from idling vehicles into classrooms (although it should be noted that the U.S. Environmental Protection Agency (EPA) has a voluntary school bus program to reduce diesel emissions) [11];
- toxic debris from construction or demolition inside occupied schools and toxic fumes from paints, glues, and new carpets [12];
- schools located in former commercial spaces, on unremediated brownfields, or on or near Superfund sites [13];
- use of toxic and explosive products in classrooms or storage of these products in schools (although the EPA has a small, voluntary school chemical clean-out program) [14];
- chemical spills or misuses that have closed schools and sent children to local emergency rooms [15];
- outbreaks of infectious diseases [16]; and
- air toxics from nearby sources such as industries or highways [17].

Federal or state programs have directed schools to deal with asbestos [18], lead in water or paint [19], underground storage tanks [20], and radon [21].

Nevertheless, not all of these problems are resolved, and there are a myriad of other problems that need to be addressed: indoor air quality (IAQ) problems, water damage (with resulting mold and bacterial growths as well as deterioration of building materials), carbon monoxide, persistent organic pollutants, inadequate sanitation and ventilation, chemical mismanagement, and poor lighting and noise controls. Shendell et al. reviewed the available science and potential exposures that these factors present [22]. It should be noted that there is no federal mandate to remove asbestos or radon or lead from schools and no mandate on testing and remediating school drinking water. No governmental agency—federal, state or local—regulates indoor air pollutants, with the exception of laws pertaining to smoking in public places; some states have enacted laws on IAQ in schools that direct districts to implement elements of the U.S. EPA's IAQ Tools for Schools voluntary protocol for good IAQ [23]. However, the U.S. EPA has de-funded its IAQ Tools for Schools grants programs, reduced staffing in 2012, and reduced funds for other schools-focused voluntary programs, creating a potential challenge to implementation. Ironically, the Institute of Medicine issued a report in 2011 finding that indoor environments are already damaging health and learning, and that exposures indoors may be 100 to 1,000 times more intense than outdoor exposures [24].

FORMULATING PUBLIC POLICY RELATED TO SCHOOLS IN THE UNITED STATES

The processes for formulation of laws and policies for schools at the national, state, or local levels are different from the processes for the formulation of most other policies. There is a complex network of laws and regulations at all three levels of government [25]. The U.S. Constitution leaves the responsibility for education to the states. Since 1980, however, there has been a Department of Education at the federal level whose primary foci are in supporting state and local educational quality, fostering achievement standards, and promoting and enforcing educational services and access for children with identified disabilities. Neither the federal Department of Education nor the federal Centers for Disease Control and Prevention (CDC), however, has the authority to regulate children's health and safety issues in schools [20]. The EPA has been authorized by Congress to create federal guidelines on specific school environmental factors and to offer voluntary grants to states to accelerate healthy school environments [26].

Nominally, states are responsible for providing public education to their citizens. Historically they have delegated much of that responsibility to local school districts [20]. There is no single system of governance for state educational systems. The National Association of State Boards of Education describes at least four models of state education governance, and exceptions to the models [27]. Therefore, it is impossible to generalize about the control of education. Moreover, environmental health issues may be addressed by the state's environment, health, energy, agriculture, or labor department, and sometimes by its education department. Individuals and organizations should acquaint themselves with the situation in their own states. With the exception of implementing state-wide immunization requirements, standardized testing, and the conduct of education, state departments of education do not function as regulatory agencies. They may have some authority to close local schools which are academically low-performing or in cases of certain emergencies [28]. Some may have specific policies or regulations that apply to facilities.

In most cities and counties around the country, schools are directed by a local board of education. Local school board members are elected independently and independent school boards have taxing authority. School boards are often independent of city or county councils and local chief executives; dependent boards report to their county or city officials.

Thus it can be a district-by-district and a state-by-state challenge to determine how to ensure that all schools, public and private, provide healthy indoor environments—in other words, are clean, dry, and quiet with good indoor air quality and thermal comfort and well-maintained systems, as recommended by the National Research Council's Committee to Review and Assess the Health and Productivity Benefits of Green Schools [29].

Because the federal government has not had the authority to regulate most environmental issues in schools, it has created multiple voluntary programs to assist schools. EPA's Healthy School Environments Assessment Tool (HealthySEAT) is a relatively new voluntary tool designed to help states and large districts assess and rate individual buildings for priority actions and repairs. It offers EPA and Occupational Safety and Health Administration (OSHA) guidance and regulations on multiple environmental factors: hazardous waste, hazardous materials, non-hazardous waste, chemical management, water, pest control, energy, mold /moisture, UV radiation, outdoor air pollution, and renovation/ construction [30]. The customizable tool:

1. includes a database file to manage all aspects of a self-assessment program;
2. includes a comprehensive and customizable sample checklist for environmental hazards and compliance;
3. fully integrates all of EPA's programs for schools; and
4. includes information on health, safety, and injury prevention programs of all other pertinent federal agencies.

The cost of state and local implementation is a barrier for this non-mandated, but highly, useful tool.

Another voluntary tool is the National Institute of Occupational Safety and Health's (NIOSH) "Safety Checklist Program for Schools," which helps school administrators, coordinators, and teachers comply with federal or state OSHA regulations. NIOSH's "Safety Checklist" focuses on classrooms, shops, and laboratories in career and technical education settings [31]. It should be noted that NIOSH focuses only on the health of adults in a workplace. It has no authority to make recommendations for protecting children who are in the same building, and its recommendations for the adults may or may not be protective of the children.

There has been no independent analysis of HealthySEAT or NIOSH's "Safety Checklist Program for Schools" to demonstrate that they are effective in changing behavior of facilities management personnel or other school personnel.

INDOOR AIR QUALITY

IAQ can be affected by external and internal sources of air pollutants. Because school buildings are generally quite old, they may have windows that are broken or that do not fit well in their casings. This may actually lead to more air flow, as compared to a tight, sealed building without operable windows. But it can also lead to the intrusion of unfiltered outdoor air pollutants and allergens—oxides of sulfur, oxides of nitrogen, particulate matter (PM_{10} and $PM_{2.5}$), air toxics, and tree and grass pollens—into the school building. Air pollutants are increased when diesel trucks or buses idle next to the air intake for the buildings heating, ventilation, and air conditioning (HVAC) systems, so that exhaust materials are sucked into the school building.

School buildings, both old and new, can have problems with dampness. This can occur as a result of building materials that have been water-damaged during construction, rain incursion through ill-fitting or damaged windows, leaks from the roof and through the floors, leaks from pipes and HVAC systems, flooding, or seepage from groundwater. The presence of excess moisture or relative high humidity indoors can lead to mold and bacterial growth and the degradation of building materials. Some of the chemicals released from the molds, bacteria, and building materials are allergens, irritants, or toxins. The presence of these and other pollutants in the air can lead to multiple health symptoms and complaints among occupants. These complaints may be diagnosed as sick building syndrome or building-related illness, two separate but related conditions. There have been numerous reports of sick building syndrome in schools [32, 33].

Off-gassing of volatile organic compounds (VOCs) from building materials or maintenance and instructional activities contribute to indoor air pollution in schools. This can include formaldehyde [34] from plywood and other volatiles from markers, from glue used under carpets, and from cleaning materials, as well as from instructional products and personal care products. VOCs can be irritants and toxins. Vapor intrusion from underground plumes of chemicals or from contamination of ground water can also be a source of VOCs in schools.

Allergens are present in the indoor air of schools [35]. Some migrate into buildings from the outside, such as tree, grass, and other pollens. In addition, animal dander can be brought into schools on the clothing of children and adults or when pets are kept in classrooms. The allergens can exacerbate allergic symptoms, including asthma, in sensitized children and adults.

Classroom ventilation is frequently inadequate, which can result in unacceptably high levels of CO_2, which can adversely affect both teacher and student performance. The American Society of Heating, Refrigerating and Air-Conditioning Engineers (ASHRAE) recommends a minimum ventilation rate of 8 liters/second/person for classrooms. This ventilation level is frequently not achieved. ASHRAE also sets a standard for CO_2 of 1,000 ppm in classrooms. Studies have shown statistically significant correlations between clinical symptoms of headaches, dizziness, tiredness, difficulties concentrating, unpleasant odor, and high CO_2 concentrations (1,500 to 4,000 ppm compared with concentrations below 1,500 ppm) [36, 37].

Although there are no standards for IAQ in schools, it is one of the few areas where the federal government has been active in promoting voluntarily programs. The U.S. EPA created the IAQ Tools for Schools program [38] in the mid-1990s and since that time has funded extensive nationwide outreach and an annual conference. This program provides guidance for do-it-yourself promotion of indoor air quality in schools. Based on the self-reported School Health Policies and Program Study, it is estimated that over 51 percent of schools (60,000 schools) in the United States have an IAQ management plan, with 85 percent of those schools reporting that their plans are based on the IAQ Tools for Schools model. It is also estimated that about two-thirds of those schools, or 38,000 schools, have effective IAQ management plans [39]. The EPA has not, however, required schools using EPA-funded technical assistance to track or report child health or learning improvements following IAQ interventions [40].

LIGHTING

Children require adequate lighting to be able to perform well in school. Many schools, however, have reported inadequate lighting, and many more have facilities that were never designed to "harvest" natural daylight into learning spaces. This is one instance where old buildings, such as those built at the turn of the last century and relied on high ceilings and tall, operable windows to provide natural daylight and ventilation, may be better. Early findings suggest that when children work in daylight or under full spectrum artificial light (light that mimics daylight), they have higher test scores and better behavior, and are healthier [41, 42].

PESTICIDES

School buildings, especially those with poor maintenance, have the potential for pest infestations because they offer moisture, food, and places to nest. For example, schools often serve meals and snacks in classrooms; children and adults may bring food to school that is kept in desks, lockers, or teachers' lounges. The books and other educational materials may also provide nutrients and habitat for pests. When pests are present, schools often mistakenly request routine application of pesticides as the primary means of control. Herbicides are also used on school grounds to control weeds. Because pesticides are designed to kill or repel rodents (rodenticides), insects (insecticides), and certain plants and fungi (herbicides and fungicides), they also have the potential to be toxic to children and adults. They can cause both acute and chronic symptoms [43]. Exposure to some pesticides on a chronic basis is associated with abnormal brain development [44]. More than three dozen states have enacted laws to restrict pesticide use in or around schools and to encourage natural control methods over more expensive routine chemical applications [44, 46].

NOISE

Noise is any unwanted, extraneous sound. Sources contributing to noise in the classroom include outside sounds from traffic, construction, and the playground as well as inside sounds from other classrooms; audio, video and computer equipment; and lighting ballasts and dimmers. Noise levels greater than 60 dBA can interfere with cognitive activities. In order to learn well, children require better acoustic quality than adults in classrooms [47]. Good speech recognition is necessary for optimal comprehension and learning during language and reading acquisition [48].

PROBLEMS OF UNKNOWN ETIOLOGY THAT MAY BE RELATED TO THE SCHOOL ENVIRONMENT

Children may develop illnesses in schools that are of unknown etiology, but may be related to their environment. For example, the CDC reported on schoolchildren in 27 states who developed noncontagious rashes at school. These children were in approximately 110 elementary, middle, and high schools. The rash was generally transient and not associated with many other symptoms. Gathering data about the extent of the problem—for example, whether children in other schools in the nation were involved—was impossible. The Healthy Schools Network, in cooperation with the American Public Health Association, the Natural Resources Defense Council, the Children's Environmental Health Network, and Beyond Pesticides requested that CDC report to Congress on its findings and on how to develop a system to establish a baseline for children's health at school [49]. No such report was ever invited by Congress.

OVERWHELMING CONTAMINATION OF SCHOOL BUILDINGS IN DISASTERS

During disasters such as hurricanes, floods, earthquakes, or terrorist events, school buildings can be used as community shelters or can be overwhelmingly contaminated with environmental hazards. Hazards can occur, for example, when floodwaters bring not only moisture leading to mold growth, but also hydrocarbons from fuel tanks or pesticides and fertilizers from farm fields. Contaminated floodwater from inundated local Superfund sites, human and animal wastes from overwhelmed sewer systems and breeched containment ponds, and other materials from upstream industrial sites can also spread contamination. Another example of overwhelming contamination occurred with the inundation of seven public schools and other buildings in the World Trade Center impact zone by air pollutants after the buildings collapsed on September 11, 2001, as documented in *Schools of Ground Zero* [50]. This dust contained asbestos, lead, and other respirable particles [50]. During the recovery period, concerns were also raised about elevated levels of CO_2, volatile organic compounds, and polychlorinated biphenyls [51]. The case dramatically underscores the lack of any system for children: There was a lack of accessible and timely information about actual contaminants, of information about risks associated with exposures specifically of this nature, of federal or state guidelines on "building clearances" for children, and of monitoring and reporting of children's health complaints.

NIOSH prepared a report on adults at schools near Ground Zero showing the onset of new diseases [52], but no agency prepared a report on schoolchildren occupying the same facilities. *Schools of Ground Zero* is the only child-centered and peer-reviewed contemporaneous account of the evacuations and contamination ever done; a take-home survey conducted with parents also indicated new illnesses among elementary-age schoolchildren.

DIFFERENCES BETWEEN PROTECTION OF CHILDREN AND PROTECTION OF ADULTS IN SCHOOLS

Private-sector workers are afforded some protection from workplace hazards by the Occupational Safety and Health Act of 1970 [53]. Public-sector workers, such as school employees, are either covered by their state Occupational Safety and Health programs (in 25 states) or are not covered at all [54]. The Occupational Safety and Health Act was developed, however, to protect the proverbial 160-pound white male industrial worker, not kindergartners or their teachers, and especially not women of child-bearing age.

Member supports are available for union members, and community support services are available to other employees that aid and abet the effective implementation of specific OSHA laws and regulations. In addition, worksite negotiations can protect employees. These related regulations or ancillary or support services, which are not available to children, include:

- local union bargaining units;
- union health and safety expertise, centrally and sometimes regionally;

- training about environmental, health, and safety issues (supported by health or labor department grants or union dues);
- in some states, department of health-funded occupational health clinics for employees with work-related concerns (in other states, private occupational health clinics may be available);
- in some states, free-standing regional nonprofit committees for occupational safety and health;
- state departments of labor;
- Occupational Safety and Health Administration–National Institute of Occupational Safety and Health;
- worker's compensation for illness or injury on the job;
- state right-to-know laws for employees or the right to form health and safety committees;
- the ability to accumulate and use sick leave or to call in a "substitute" for a day or for an extended absence;
- the ability to switch job locations; and
- for some school jobs, the ability to work part-time or to carry out part of the job from home [41, 55, 56].

Yet, even in situations where adult employees may recognize and ask about a health problem related to an exposure at work or in school, much of the effort to try to demonstrate that link and to get the situation resolved falls on the individual employee. OSHA also does not necessarily protect workers from commonly encountered indoor environmental hazards—such as indoor air or molds or the intrusion of outdoor pollutants—that are not specifically linked to an employee's job of handling hazardous materials or engaging in hazardous work activities, such as operating heavy equipment, construction, or assembly-line work.

Schools are also extremely reluctant to recognize that children could be affected by the same health hazards that are affecting adults in the building. New York State has a network of state-funded occupational health clinics that adults can access. These are not, however, set up to respond to queries regarding children. Such clinics have the capability to do on-site evaluations, but they must obtain permission from the schools to do so [41, 55, 57]. There are no programs anywhere in the country specifically authorized, trained, and staffed to do health hazard evaluations for children in child care centers or schools, despite the fact that the adults in those workplaces have continuing occupational safety and health concerns.

It is said that two major advantages that parents have in dealing with school environmental issues are that their jobs are not on the line and that they can readily communicate with community and with media. It is also said that children may have actionable rights under federal law for an "accessible" facility and program, for example, under Section 504 of the Rehabilitation Act, Americans with Disabilities Act, or Individual with Disabilities Education Act. In turn, parents have countered, especially those with children with disabilities and other special needs, that they are utterly dependent on negotiating with the local school district to fulfill its obligations under federal law for the education of children with disabilities, including health impairments and are, therefore, reluctant to upset the negotiations with additional requests for a healthy environment [58].

The lack of formal systems to protect children shortchanges all parties. As a result, parents must fall back on their own informal resources if they suspect their children are having environment-related health problems due to the school environment. Schools are deprived of independent assessments that take their most vulnerable occupants, and most important output, into account. Skilled individuals appropriate to the need, are simply not trained and available, nor are agency authorizations in place. Most primary health care offices and/or pediatricians do not have the knowledge necessary to evaluate the situations [59-61]. Moreover, the evaluation of school-related environmental health problems requires a multidisciplinary approach. A physician should evaluate the individuals involved, and industrial hygienists with knowledge about how children interact with their environment and buildings, along with a working knowledge of relevant federal, state, and city laws and regulations or best practices. Other specialists with knowledge of building sciences, chemical policies, or about HVAC systems or other systems may also be needed. Parents need formal backup and ongoing advice. As presently organized, of course, the school must be willing to invite an onsite investigation that benefits children.

DATA COLLECTION

The example about the rash illnesses given above indicates some of the issues around data collection. There is no systematic method for collecting health data on children in schools. Neither the CDC nor the National Center for Education Statistics of the U.S. Department of Education collects information specifically related to school environmental health issues.

The Environmental Health Tracking Program of the CDC also does not provide a means to collect data about the health of children in schools. First, it was designed to compare existing health and environmental data bases; and, second, there are no databases on school environmental health. With the exception of efforts in Florida, Massachusetts, Connecticut, and California, where some information about asthma was collected [62], all attempts to collect environmental public health tracking data from schools have been stymied by the Family Education Rights and Privacy Act (FERPA). FERPA limits access to educational data unless there is express permission for parents, guardians, or the child (if old enough). By lumping school health data with other educational information,

FERPA has made schoolchildren's health data inaccessible for public health research purposes [63].

School nurses, unfortunately, also are not a reliable source of environmental information related to children. First, they may not be permitted to share information or to speak with parents about building conditions impacting children. Second, school nurses are not mandated staff positions. And third, there is no standardized system into which school nurses can report data. One small informal survey, which should be replicated, raised serious concerns about whether school nurses can or would participate, given their lack of independence and stated job retaliation fears [64].

Pediatric Environmental Health Specialty Units (PEHSUs) were created about a decade ago, co-funded through The Association of Occupational and Environmental Clinics (AOEC) by the EPA and the CDC [65]. There is no uniform approach or knowledge base on school-based problems among the PEHSUs. By design, the PEHSUs are reactive rather than proactive. Some of the PEHSUs, however, have taken a proactive approach to glaring problems in their home communities. Therefore, while PEHSUs are an educational resource about children's vulnerabilities, they are not a source of data about children's environmental health in schools.

RECOMMENDATIONS

In the current world, there are numerous environmental health hazards that can affect the health of school personnel and schoolchildren. Though the laws, regulations, policies, and programs that protect adults are not as comprehensive or as effective as they could be, such laws, regulations, and policies are utterly nonexistent for children. The publicly supported environmental public health programs to serve children and their families are woefully inadequate.

Based on these findings, we recommend that children in child care centers and schools through grade 12 have access to a range of environmental public health services similar to, but independent of, the array of research, training, information, support, and clinical services available to protect adults in their workplaces. One public health agency at the federal level, advised by EPA, child environmental health advocates, and experienced parents, must be authorized and funded to establish a program. This program should be independent of the educational system at the state and local levels. The program might include some or all of the following key elements:

1. That a data collection system for school environmental health problems be established. Such a model school health tracking data collection system should describe what parameters should be tracked, what type of database

should be used, who should do the data entry, where the data should go, and how it should be made public.

2. That an environmental public health tracking system be implemented in at least sentinel school systems throughout the country. (See below for recommendations about overcoming barriers to implementing environmental public health tracking in schools.)
3. That federal agencies develop a coordinated federal strategy for the states to help their schools rapidly improve facility design, construction, and maintenance, as well as set up programs to test for and remediate hazards and to phase in safer products.
4. That adequate research be funded, conducted, and published so that standards for indoor environmental quality can be promulgated that are appropriate to children's higher respiration rates and enhanced vulnerability to toxins.
5. That, where adequate information currently exists, states develop enforceable regulations regarding indoor environmental quality for schools; and that, as new information is developed, those regulations be updated. An agency other than the education agency should be responsible for oversight and enforcements.
6. That federal and state agencies provide direction to and supplementary funding for the PEHSUs so that they can be staffed and personnel specifically trained to address environmental health risks in child care centers and schools.
7. That PEHSUs be authorized to facilitate on-site inspections of child care centers and schools when necessary.
8. That a review of school closures that have been taken for health and safety reasons be published and used to determine if current laws and regulations are sufficient for protection of public health or need to be amended or replaced.
9. That EPA regional offices be charged with and funded to adapt the HealthySEAT guidelines for state-by-state use. This would allow health care providers, PEHSUs, parents, and communities to have access to relevant federal, state, and local laws as well as regulations and best practices related to environmental health in schools.
10. That a meeting be convened between representatives of the Department of Health and Human Services (National Institutes of Health, CDC) and the Department of Education, the Department of Justice, outside legal experts, and child health advocates to discuss the issue of research and data collection in and about schools and about schoolchildren. This meeting should review the barriers that FERPA represents in the context of environmental public health tracking and research on school environmental health.

NOTES

1. P. S. Guzelian, C. J. Henry, and S. S. Olin (eds.), *Similarities and Differences between Children and Adults: Implications for Risk Assessment* (Washington, DC: ILSI Press, 1992).
2. S. G. Selevan, C. A. Kimmel, and P. Mendola, "Identifying Critical Windows of Exposure for Children's Health," *Environmental Health Perspectives* 108(3) suppl. (2000): 451-455, http://www.crossref.org/guestquery/
3. R. L. Brent and M. Weitzman, "The Current State of Knowledge about the Effects, Risks, and Science of Children's Environmental Exposures," *Pediatrics* 113-114 suppl. (2004): 1158-1166.
4. U.S. Department of Education, National Center for Education Statistics, *Digest of Education Statistics, 2010*, April 5, 2011.
5. Government Accounting Office, *School Facilities: Condition of America's Schools* (GAO/HEHS-95-61, February 1, 1995), http://www.gao.gov/archive/1995/he95061.pdf (accessed July 20, 2009).
6. U.S. Department of Education. *The Condition of Education 2000* (Report NCES 2000-062). (Washington, DC: National Center for Education Statistics, 2000).
7. Center for Health, Environment, and Justice, "Poisoned Schools: Invisible Threats, Visible Actions," https://www.chej.org/publications/health.htm (accessed November 20, 2009).
8. Agency for Toxic Substances and Disease Registry with U.S. EPA and Morehouse School of Medicine Regional Research Center for Minority Health (oral presentation at American Public Health Association, October 2001).
9. L. Lewis et al., *Condition of America's Public School Facilities: 1999* (National Center for Education Statistics, U.S. Department of Education, Office of Educational Research and Improvement), NCES 2000-032, 2000, http://nces.ed.gov/pubs2000/2000032.pdf (accessed July 30, 2009).
10. S. E. Jones, R. Axelrad, and W. A. Wattgney, "Healthy and Safe School Environment. Part II. Physical School Environment: Results from the School Health Policies and Program Study 2006," *Journal of School Health* 77 (2007): 544-556.
11. U.S. Environmental Protection Agency, "Clean School Bus USA," http://www.epa.gov/cleanschoolbus/ (accessed July 20, 2009).
12. U.S. Environmental Protection Agency, "IAQ Design Tools for Schools (DTfS): Construction," http://www.epa.gov/iaq/schooldesign/construction.html (accessed July 20, 2009).
13. B. D. Brewer et al., "Characteristics of Schools on or near Hazardous Waste Sites in Brownfields Communities" (Abstract 23956), Annual Meeting, American Public Health Association, Atlanta, GA, October 21-25, 2001, http://apha.confex.com/apha/129am/techprogram/paper_23956.htm (accessed July 20, 2009).
14. U.S. Environmental Protection Agency, "Healthy School Environment Resources: On-Site Chemical Management," http://cfpub.epa.gov/schools/top_sub.cfm?t_id=361&s_id=364 (accessed July 24, 2009).
15. Centers for Disease Control and Prevention, "Hazardous Substances Emergency Events Surveillance," http://www.atsdr.cdc.gov/HS/HSEES/ (accessed July 20, 2009).

16. Anonymous, "Update: Measles—United States, January-July 2008," *Morbidity & Mortality Weekly Report* 57 (2008): 893-896.
17. U.S. Environmental Protection Agency, "Assessing Outdoor Air Near Schools," http://www.epa.gov/schoolair/ (accessed July 20, 2009).
18. U.S. Environmental Protection Agency, "Asbestos in Schools," http://www.epa.gov/asbestos/pubs/asbestos_in_schools.html (accessed July 27, 2009).
19. U.S. Environmental Protection Agency, "Drinking Water in Schools and Child Care Facilities," http://www.epa.gov/safewater/schools (accessed July 27, 2009).
20. U.S. Environmental Protection Agency, "Underground Storage Tanks," http://www.epa.gov/swerust1/ (accessed July 27, 2009).
21. U.S. Environmental Protection Agency, "Radon in Schools (2nd Ed.)," http://www.epa.gov/radon/pubs/schoolrn.html (accessed July 27, 2009).
22. D. G. Shendell, C. Barnett, and S. Boese, "Science-Based Recommendations to Prevent or Reduce Potential Exposure to Biological, Chemical, and Physical Agents in Schools," *Journal of School Health* 74 (2004): 390-397.
23. Environmental Law Institute, "Database of State Indoor Air Quality Laws," http://www.eli.org/Program_Areas/iaq_databases.cfm, (accessed July 20, 2009).
24. Institute of Medicine of the National Academies, *Climate Change, the Indoor Environment and Health* (Washington, DC: The National Academies Press, 2011).
25. Centers for Division Control and Prevention Division of Adolescent and School Health, "A CDC Review of School Laws and Policies Concerning Child and Adolescent Health," *Journal of School Health* 78 (2008): 69-128.
26. U.S. Department of Energy, "The Energy Independence and Security Act of 2007, Section 504," http://www1.eere.energy.gov/femp/regulations/eisa.html#top (accessed July 30, 2009).
27. National Association of State Boards of Education, "2009 State Education Governance Models," http://nasbe.org/index.php/file-repository/func-startdown/960/ (accessed November 2, 2009).
28. J. G. Hodge, D. Bhattacharya, and J. Gray, *Legal Preparedness for School Closures in Response to Pandemic Influenza and Other Emergencies: A Review and Report* (submitted to the U.S. Centers for Disease Control and Prevention, Center for Law and the Public's Health, Baltimore, Maryland) http://www2a.cdc.gov/phlp/docs/Legal%20Preparedness%20for%20School%20Closures%20in%20Response%20to%20Pandemic%20Influenza.pdf (accessed July 24, 2009).
29. National Research Council's Committee to Review and Assess the Health and Productivity Benefits of Green Schools, *Green Schools: Attributes for Health and Learning* (Washington, DC: National Academies Press, 2006).
30. U.S. Environmental Protection Agency, "Healthy School Environments Assessment Tool," http://www.epa.gov/schools/healthyseat/ (accessed July 20, 2009).
31. National Institute for Occupational Safety and Health, "Safety Checklist Program for Schools," http://www.cdc.gov/niosh/docs/2004-101/ (accessed July 27, 2009).
32. C. M. Scheel, W. C. Rosing, and A. L. Farone, "Possible Sources of Sick Building Syndrome in a Tennessee Middle School," *Archives of Environmental Health* 56 (2001): 413.
33. Institute of Medicine of the National Academies' Committee on Damp Indoor Spaces and Health, *Damp Indoor Spaces and Health*. (Washington, DC: The National Academies Press, 2004).

34. C. van Netten, "Analysis of Sources Contributing to Elevated Formaldehyde Concentrations in the Air in a New Elementary School," *Canadian Journal of Public Health (Revue Canadienne de Santé Publique)* 74 (1983): 55-59.
35. S. L. Abramson et al., "Allergens in School Settings: Results of Environmental Assessments in 3 City School Systems," *Journal of School Health* 76 (2006): 246-249.
36. A. N. Myhrvold, E. Olsen, and O. Lauridsen, "Indoor Environment in Schools—Pupils' Health and Performance in Regard to CO_2 Concentrations," Proceedings of Indoor Air '96: The 7th International Conference on Indoor Air Quality and Climate, Nagoya, Japan, July, 1996 (Vol. 4, 369-374), as quoted in J. M. Daisey, W. J. Angell, and M. G. Apte, "Indoor Air Quality, Ventilation and Health Symptoms in Schools: An Analysis of Existing Information," *Indoor Air* 13 (2003): 53-64.
37. J. M. Daisey, W. J. Angell, and M. G. Apte, "Indoor Air Quality, Ventilation and Health Symptoms in Schools: An Analysis of Existing Information," *Indoor Air* 13 (2003): 53-64.
38. U.S. Environmental Protection Agency, "Tools for Schools Program," http://www.epa.gov/iaq/schools/ (accessed July 20, 2009).
39. U.S. Centers for Disease Control and Prevention, *School Health Policies and Programs Study 2006. Physical School Environment*, 2006, http://www.cdc.gov/HealthyYouth/shpps/2006/factsheets/pdf/FS_PhysicalSchoolEnvironment_SHPPS2006.pdf (accessed July 30, 2009).
40. U.S. Environmental Protection Agency, *Letter to the U.S. EPA Administrator from the Federal Advisory Committee at the EPA Office of Children's Health Protection*, 2002, http://yosemite.epa.gov/ochp/ochpweb.nsf/content/522002.htm/$file/522002.pdf (accessed July 20, 2009).
41. Healthy Schools Network, Inc., *Healthy Schools Network Guide: Better Lighting for Healthier Students*, [no date], http://www.healthyschools.org/downloads/Lighting_Guide.pdf (accessed July 20, 2009).
42. B. Erwine, "Lighting," in *Safe and Healthy School Environments*, eds. H. Frumkin, R. Geller, I. L. Rubin, and J. Nodvin, 20-33. (Oxford: Oxford University Press, 2006).
43. U.S. Environmental Protection Agency, "Recognition and Management of Pesticide Poisonings," http://www.epa.gov/opp00001/safety/healthcare/handbook/handbook.htm (accessed July 20, 2009).
44. B. Weiss, S. Amler, and R. W. Amler, "Pesticides," *Pediatrics* 113 (2004): 1030-1036.
45. K. Owens and J. Feldman, (Beyond Pesticides/National Coalition Against the Misuse of Pesticides), *The Schooling of State Pesticide Laws—2002 Update: A Review of State Pesticide Laws Regarding Schools*, 2002, http://www.beyondpesticides.org/schools/publications/School_report_update_2002.pdf (accessed July 27, 2009).
46. L. Kann, N. D. Brener, and H. Wechsler, "Overview and Summary: School Health Policies and Programs Study 2006," *Journal of School Health* 77 (2007): 385-397.
47. L. E. Maxwell, "Noise" in *Safe and Healthy School Environments*, ed. H. Frumkin, R. Geller, I. L. Rubin, and J. Nodvin, 34-45. (Oxford: Oxford University Press, 2006).
48. D. G. Shendell, C. Barnett, and S. Boese, "Science-Based Recommendations to Prevent or Reduce Potential Exposure to Biological, Chemical, and Physical Agents in Schools," *Journal of School Health* 74 (2004): 390-394.
49. Anonymous, "Update: Rashes among Schoolchildren—27 States, October 4, 2001-June 3, 2002," *Morbidity & Mortality Weekly Report* 51 (2002): 524-527.

50. S. Bartlett and J. Petrarca, *Schools of Ground Zero: Early Lessons Learned in Children's Environmental Health* (Washington, DC: American Public Health Association, 2002).
51. Pediatric Environmental Health Specialty Unit, Mount Sinai Medical Center, *World Trade Center Fact Sheets*, http://www.mountsinai.org/Research/Centers%20Laboratories%20and%20Programs/Pediatric%20Environmental%20Health%20Specialty%20Unit/Overview/Fact%20Sheets (accessed July 24, 2009).
52. National Institute for Occupational Safety and Health, *NIOSH Health Hazard Evaluation Report (HETA #2002-0090; 2002-0096; 2002-0101-3028: Buildings in the Vicinity of the World Trade Center, New York)*, http://www.cdc.gov/niosh/hhe/reports/pdfs/2002-0101-3028.pdf (accessed July 24, 2009).
53. U.S. Department of Labor, Occupational Safety and Health Administration, "Occupational Safety and Health Act of 1970," http://www.osha.gov/pls/oshaweb/owasrch.search_form?p_doc_type=oshact (accessed July 20, 2009).
54. U.S. Department of Labor, Occupational Safety and Health Administration, "State Occupational Safety and Health Plans," http://www.osha.gov/dcsp/osp/index.html (accessed July 30, 2009).
55. G. Siwinski (Industrial Hygienist, New York State Central New York Occupational Health Clinic, Syracuse, NY), personal communication, January 2005.
56. D. Newman (Industrial Hygienist, New York Committee for Occupational Safety and Health), personal communication, February 2005.
57. D. Newman (Industrial Hygienist, New York Committee for Occupational Safety and Health) in discussion with author, February 2005.
58. Healthy Schools Network, Inc., *Who's in Charge of Protecting Children's Health at Schools?*, 2005, http://www.healthyschools.org/documents/WhosInCharge.pdf (accessed July 30, 2009).
59. J. R. Roberts and B. A. Gitterman, "Pediatric Environmental Health Education: A Survey of U.S. Pediatric Residency Programs," *Ambulatory Pediatrics* 3 (2003): 57-59.
60. L. Trasande et al., "The Environment in Pediatric Practice: A Study of New York Pediatricians' Attitudes, Beliefs, and Practices towards Children's Environmental Health," *Journal of Urban Health* 83 (2006): 760-772.
61. L. Trasande, N. Graber, and P. J. Landrigan, "Does New York State Need a System of Referral Centers for Children with Environmental Health Concerns?", Pediatric Academic Societies Meeting, Washington, DC, 2005.
62. L. Hines (National Center for Environmental Health, Centers for Disease Control and Prevention), personal communication, July 08, 2009.
63. J. G. Hodge and L. F. Wiley, "An Assessment of Legal Issues Concerning Public Health Disclosures Pursuant to Proposed Rulemaking re: The Family Education Rights and Privacy Act (FERPA), Council of State and Territorial Epidemiologists," 2008, http://www.cste.org/dnn/LinkClick.aspx?fileticket=hXbae9TZBJg%3D&tabid=184&mid=733 (accessed July 24, 2009).
64. New York State Association of School Nurses with Healthy Schools Network, *What School Nurses Know: We Need New Laws to Clean-up Schools*, May 2000.
65. J. A. Paulson et al., "Development of the Pediatric Environmental Health Specialty Unit Network: The North American Experience," *American Journal of Public Health* (in press).

CHAPTER 2

Who's Sick at School: Linking Poor School Conditions and Health Disparities for Boston's Children

Tolle Graham, Jean Zotter, and Marlene Camacho

We know what the problem is and we have the findings, so why does it take so long to get repairs done? It should be about the health of our children, yet why does it take so long? The money should be in the budget to fix our schools."

– *Mary White, BUAC Parent Leader, parent of two BPS students, on fixing our school buildings*

A recent review of student asthma rates and environmental audits of school buildings suggests that schools with poor indoor air quality have higher-than-average rates of asthma. Many Boston Public School (BPS) children and staff are learning and working in poor indoor environmental conditions that not only can exacerbate asthma, but also lead to other problems ranging from allergies and sinus infections to adverse academic performance [1]. The Boston Urban Asthma Coalition (BUAC) conducted a preliminary analysis of 2004-05 childhood asthma rates for BPS students and compared them to the 2004-05 environmental audits of the top 10 schools with environmental problems. This analysis suggests that schools with the highest rates of leaks, mold, and pest infestations also have higher-than-average asthma rates for children.

PROBLEM

Asthma is a condition in which the airways in the lung constrict and become inflamed. It can result in loss of breath and loss of life. An asthma attack can be precipitated by exposure to allergens such as mold or pests, irritants, or cold temperature. Asthma is the leading cause of school absenteeism due to chronic illness, accounting for more than 12 million missed school days per year [2]. Nationally, inequities in health conditions, such as asthma, together may account for as much as a quarter of the racial gap in school readiness [3]. The cause or causes of asthma are still unclear although research has found that exposure to pests, molds, diesel exhaust, and environmental tobacco smoke play key roles in asthma's development and exacerbation.

Childhood asthma is a major public health concern for the City of Boston and one that disproportionately impacts children of color. Asthma is the number one chronic condition treated in Boston Public Schools. Between 7% and 12% of the BPS student body in grades K–8 have asthma [4], and this number may be an underestimate of the extent of the problem for Boston's children as other local studies have found much higher childhood asthma rates for Boston's children [5]. Boston has higher childhood asthma hospitalization rates than the rest of the state, with children of color having much higher rates [6]. Latino and Black children suffer from asthma more than Boston's White children do [7].

As Boston sets forth to tackle health disparities, addressing environmental factors that make asthma worse should be a top priority. Students are primarily children of color, with 74% qualifying for free or reduced-rate meals [8]. Many BPS families have no choice to send their children to a healthier school because of their economic situation. For many BPS students and their families, advocating for improved environmental conditions is their only recourse.

Poor school environmental conditions are one of many components that affect a child's asthma. Housing conditions, outdoor air quality, and environmental tobacco smoke are among other factors that also affect a child's health. Sixty-three percent of the housing in Boston was built before 1950 and 75% was built before the lead paint laws passed (1978). Twenty-five percent of the homes receive federal or state subsidies to charge below fair-market rate. Many Boston families rent their apartments (approximately 63% of Boston residents) and lack affordable housing options (Boston ranks 48th in affordable housing), and so often have little control over housing conditions and little influence over the actions of their landlord. In Boston, air toxics exceed by 128 times the Environmental Protection Agency's (EPA) safe level of carcinogen in the air [9]. School conditions are only part of the picture, but with children spending increasingly long hours in school buildings, school conditions play an important role in creating health disparities in asthma. It's a role that should not be ignored.

> I know from my own experience in our old apartment that certain asthma triggers such as carpeting sent me to the emergency room many times with my daughter. As a BUAC Parent Leader in the Strengthening Voices project, I learned a lot about the asthma triggers in our schools. Now I tell other parents and teachers how important it is to speak up about the poor conditions in our schools so we can get them fixed.
>
> *– Bridget Hickson, BUAC Parent Leader, BPS Parent*

BOSTON PUBLIC SCHOOLS

BPSs are mandated by city ordinance to conduct bi-annual environmental inspections for all elementary, middle, and high schools. These inspections serve as a method of tracking the environmental status of all city public schools [10]. As part of the inspections, data regarding leaks and visible water stains, visible mold growth, overt pest signs, improper chemical storage, and repairs needed are tracked. While there are other environmental issues that were inspected, we will address these issues specifically because of their direct relationship to triggering asthma episodes. Leaks are of concern because moisture can promote mold growth as well as encourage insect or rodent infestations. Visible mold growth is important because mold and mildew are often asthma triggers. Pests are of concern for sanitation reasons as well as being sources of animal dander that can be an asthma or allergy trigger. Improper chemical storage can be an issue because toxic fumes and chemicals can aggravate asthma as well. The use of chemicals through pesticides and cleaning products has also been linked to other health problems including behavioral disabilities and damage to the nervous and immune systems [11]. Building repairs are important because they can stop a small problem from getting bigger—such as immediately fixing a leak in a ceiling could stop mold from growing later.

> One of the major concerns at the Curley is that the building needs to be pointed. We have been on a list for four years and the project always gets postponed. We have water that makes its way into the building causing leaks, paint to flake and fall on students and teachers, and dust to cover the radiators. As a result many of our students with asthma are affected—so many have poor attendance because they are out a lot and as a result their grades suffer.
>
> *– Geraldo Martinez, Principal*
> *Mary E. Curley Middle School*

RESULTS

The overall estimated asthma rate for Boston Public Schools during spring 2005 is 7.0% [12]. The rates across BPSs range from 0% to 27%; these asthma rates, however, do not include high schools [12]. Many schools had asthma rates well above the state average; in addition, inspections of the schools noted an overwhelming presence of environmental issues which contribute to the incidence of asthmatic children in schools.

Figure 1 represents the percentage of schools within the BPS system during the 2004-2005 school year that reported the presence of environmental issues such as leaks, mold, or overt pest infestation.

Looking at Figure 1, approximately 85% of BPSs reported leaks or water stains, 36% reported visible mold growth, 63% reported overt pest signs, 83% reported repairs needed, and 61% reported improper chemical storage [13].

> I got adult onset of asthma, I believe, from working in a sick school building with a roof that was leaking and [had] mold all over. I went on daily medication to deal with my breathing problems. Now, three years away from that building and working in another school, I no longer need my asthma meds. School buildings that are not maintained are a health problem for students and staff.
>
> – *Sue Trotz, Boston School Guidance Councilor*

For the 2004-2005 school year, The Harvard Kent Elementary School in Charlestown reported the highest percentage of water intrusion issues with 62.5% of rooms inspected having leaks or visible water stains [13]. The James Curley Elementary School in Jamaica Plain had the highest percentage of overt pest signs, approximately 60.7% of all rooms inspected [13]. These schools both have significant higher rates of asthma than the city average of 7% (12.25% and 10.69% respectively). While environmental problems in the school may not be responsible for the higher asthma prevalences, the presence of triggers such as mold and pests do aggravate children who have already been diagnosed with

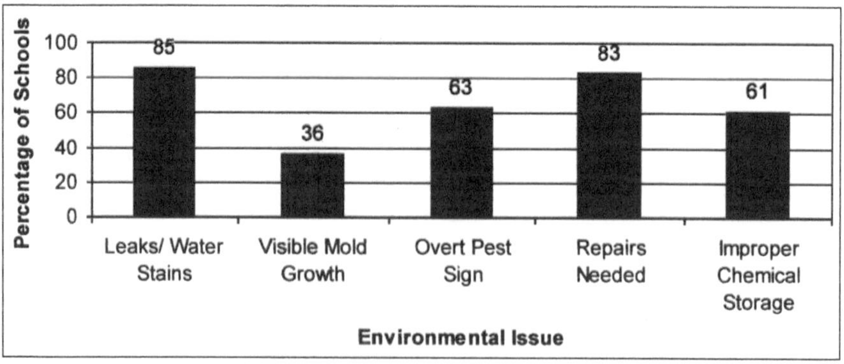

Figure 1. Percentage of Boston Public Schools with Environmental Issues, 2004-2005

asthma, increasing the incidence of asthma attacks at schools. The presence of these triggers also contributes to increased absenteeism among asthmatics and more frequent trips to the school nurse [14].

Table 1 shows the top 10 ranked schools for the categories of leaks, water stains, mold, and pests for the 2004-2005 school year. The percentages listed indicate the percentage of rooms with the presence of the environmental issue [15]. BUAC calculated the asthma rates using raw data collected by the BPS Department [16].

Further analysis of data will be required to fully assess the connection between asthma rates and environmental conditions. The Department of Public Health will soon release a report on their statewide findings on asthma rates and their link to environmental factors in school which will help further this area of research. Regardless of the link, pests and leaks are known asthma triggers that make children with asthma more sick once exposed. A child with asthma who attends a school with a 60% pest infestation rate will have difficulty learning if the pest droppings trigger his asthma.

COMMUNITY EFFORTS

To address concerns about poor school conditions and health, the BUAC and MassCOSH won compliance with a 1996 ordinance stating that Boston Public Schools must conduct bi-annual environmental inspections for all elementary, middle, and high schools in the year 2002. Another outcome of the compliance was the creation of the Healthy Schools Taskforce. The joint task force brings together parents, community and health organizations, and city councilors, BPSs, the Boston Public Health Commission to jointly resolve air quality problems, such as pests and cleaning chemicals. This task force will continue to address the issues raised by this report. However, many changes require leadership from the top. The following recommendations can only be accomplished with the support and leadership of Boston Mayor Thomas Menino.

RECOMMENDATIONS

BUAC and MassCOSH call upon the City of Boston and Mayor Menino to take immediate steps to promote a safe and healthy school environment for children and school employees by:

- Funding an independent report on the condition of the BPSs to determine what it will cost to repair and upgrade our buildings (including roofs, pointing, HVAC systems, mold remediation) and create a safe and healthy learning environment. The report should include an evaluation of the annual environmental audits and their effectiveness in improving school building maintenance and best practices for environmental safety and health.

Table 1. Top 10 Schools Ranked by Percentage of Rooms with Environmental Problems

Top 10 schools with problem	Percentage of rooms with problem	Asthma %
Leaks		
1. Harvard/Kent*	62.5	12.25
2. Mary Curley*	58.0	11.66
3. Lewis	54.2	n/a
4. Ohrenberger	53.3	n/a
5. Condon	46.0	15.54
6. Cleveland	41.3	13.34
7. Mattahunt	392.	3.71
8. Agassiz*	390	11.29
9. McKay	38.2	6.00
10. Tynan	37.2	10.70
Pests		
1. James Curley	60.7	10.69
2. Health Careers Academy	56.3	5.31
3. Hennigan	50.0	9.51
4. Harbor Elementary	48.6	12.45
5. Dearborn	41.1	16.29
6. Mary Curley	40.6	11.66
7. Taylor	40.0	5.31
8. Quincy Upper 3	38.5	n/a
9. Carter Development Center	35.0	n/a
10. Hale	33.3	10.61
Mold		
1. Quincy Upper 3*	38.5	n/a
2. West Roxbury High	28.3	n/a
3. Quincy Upper 2	17.6	n/a
4. Excel High	8.2	n/a
5. Clap Elementary	7.7	7.35
6. Fenway High	7.1	n/a
7. Beethoven	6.8	3.18
8. Harvard/Kent	6.3	12.25
9. Agassiz	5.2	11.29
10. Grew	5.1	7.84

*Schools appear on multiple "top ten" lists.

N/A, These schools either failed to report their asthma rates or are high schools which currently are not part of the asthma surveillance system.

- Validating the current asthma surveillance system and making all efforts to include all BPS children in the report, such as high school students and those students from schools with incomplete or missing reports.
- Adopting Boston's Green Building Taskforce's recommendations for building and renovating healthy high performance buildings as a model for the BPSs.
- Advocating that the Massachusetts School Building Authority adopt the MA-CHPS (healthy high-performance school design criteria) into its new regulations by July 2006.
- Committing to appropriating $200 million in capital expenditures estimated to upgrade and repair schools as necessary to create a safe, healthy environment. Building repairs and upgrades should prioritize items that result in unsafe or unhealthy conditions (for example, leaks that result in mold). The city should investigate other methods of financing these repairs by surveying other cities and states.
- Finishing the retrofit of the Boston School bus fleet to reduce diesel pollution in our neighborhoods, initiated by the school department with EPA funding in 2003.
- Pass a resolution at the next U.S. Conference of Mayors on Children's Environmental Health and School Building Conditions to promote a national dialogue and actions needed to address our aging school buildings.

> It's imperative that we get funding to fix our schools immediately. We need to do something about the leaks and the mice. Students and teachers are getting sick.
>
> –*Nia Burke, Physical Education Teacher, Boston Teachers Union*

ACKNOWLEDGMENTS

This report was written and produced by the Massachusetts Coalition for Occupational Safety and Health (MassCOSH) and the Boston Urban Asthma Coalition's (BUAC) Healthy Schools Committee with the assistance of public health intern Marlene Camacho. BUAC representatives are members of the joint City-Wide Healthy Schools Task Force which was established in 2003 with the school department and health commission to monitor the implementation of the annual environmental audits and address other environmental health and safety issues as they affect health and learning in Boston schools. This article was written in response to a request by the school department to help raise awareness in Boston about the importance of building, renovating, and maintaining safe, healthy learning spaces. BUAC believes that children with asthma are like the "canaries in the mines." When we improve our school buildings and rid them of the significant asthma triggers (mold, pests, chemicals, and fumes), we will achieve a school environment that is healthy for everyone.

MassCOSH is a non-profit organization that advocates for safe, secure jobs and healthy communities. MassCOSH coordinates the Mass Healthy Schools Network, a statewide coalition that works with parents, students, school staff, public health and environmental advocates to promote environmentally healthy and safe schools through advocacy, education, organizing, and technical assistance.

BUAC is comprised of 200 Boston residents and parents, community-based organizations, government agencies, medical professionals, and other individuals who share the common interest of improving the Boston community in order to halt the growing asthma crisis in low-income neighborhoods. The Coalition serves as a clearinghouse and network for those in the city who are committed to improving the problem of asthma in Boston. Strengthening Voices, a program of BUAC, supports parent leadership on asthma through community organizing and education. Community-led committees on Housing, Healthy Schools and Access to Quality Healthcare develop the advocacy work and activities of the coalition.

We would like to thank the following members of the BUAC Healthy Schools Committee who contributed to this report with information, statistics, and advice: Marlene Camacho, BUAC intern for this report; Jean Zotter, Director, BUAC; Nealdra Osgood, Strengthening Voices Program Director, BUAC; Mary White, BUAC Parent Leader; Bridget Hickson, BUAC Parent Leader; Davida Andelman, BUAC Steering Committee Chair, Bowdoin Street Community Health Center; Isabel Lopez, Community Labor Coordinator, MassCOSH; Tolle Graham, Healthy Schools Coordinator, MassCOSH; Lilliam Hebbert, Healthy Schools Committee member, Boston Asthma Initiative; Mary Mulvey Jacobson; Ginny Lane, retired teacher, BTU; Nancy Sullivan, Assistant Director School Health Services, Boston Public Schools; John Shea, Director of Environmental Hazards Program, Boston Public Health Commission; and Jalal Ghaemghami, Principal Toxicologist, Boston Public Health Commission. We especially want to thank Boston City Council Education Committee's co-chairs—Councilor Chuck Turner for his leadership and support in securing the annual environmental audits and Councilor John Tobin for his support for the city-wide Healthy Schools Task Force.

REFERENCES

1. M. J. Mendell, G. A. Heath. Do indoor pollutants and thermal conditions in schools influence student performance? A critical review of the literature. *Indoor Air* 2005 Feb;15(1):27-52.
2. National Center for Health Statistics. Raw Data from the National Health Interview Survey, U.S., 2003. (Analysis by the American Lung Association, Using SPSS and SUDAAN software).

3. J. Currie. Health disparities and gaps in school readiness. *Future Child.* 2005 Spring; 15(1):117-38.
4. Over the last 4 years, the asthma rate in Boston Public Schools has ranged from 12% to 7%.
5. One study found that 56% of the children in the Franklin Hill Housing Development had doctor-diagnosed asthma. D. Brugge et al., An Asthma Intervention Pilot Study in Public Housing: Lessons and Baseline Data, Engineering Solutions to Indoor Air Quality Programs Symposium, U.S. EPA 2000. In addition, the Massachusetts asthma rate for children is 12.3%, the same as the New England regional rate. It is difficult to believe that Boston has a childhood asthma rate lower than the rest of the state when our adult asthma rates exceed the state average and childhood asthma rates are traditionally higher than adult rates. Child Asthma in New England: A Report by the New England Asthma Regional Council. January 2004. www.asthmaregionalcouncil.org. *Health of Boston,* 2005, Boston Public Health Commission, Research and Technical Services, Boston, MA 02118.
6. *Health of Boston,* 2005. Boston's children under the age of 5 experience the highest hospitalization rates at 8.9 per 1,000—four times the Massachusetts rate.
7. Ibid. In 2004, Black children under the age of 5 had the highest asthma hospitalization rate of 10.7 per 1,000 and Latino children under the age of 5 had 8.6 per 1,000 while White children of the same age had a rate of 2 per 1,000.
8. Boston Public Schools website: www. http://boston.k12.ma.us/
9. National Resources Defense Council. http://www.nrdc.org/air/pollution/cep/cbos.asp
10. The inspections began in 2002 after a city council hearing initiated by City Councilor Charles Turner and the Boston Urban Asthma Coalition. City ordinance mandates that each school receive bi-annual inspections for air quality problems. As of 2003, four inspections per school have been conducted. The most recent results can be found on the BPS website: www.http://boston.k12.ma.us/
11. Boston Urban Asthma Coalition, MassCOSH, Boston Public Health Commission, and Boston Public Schools. Integrated Pest Management Promoting Healthier and Pest-Free Schools.
12. Boston Public Schools. Raw Data collected from Pediatric Asthma Surveillance (K–8) Spring 2005.
13. Boston Public Schools. School Environmental Inspection Report. 2005.
14. S. A. Moonie, D. A. Sterling, L. Figgs, M. Castro. Asthma status and severity affects missed school days. *Journal of School Health*. 2006 Jan;76(1):18-24.
15. Boston Public Schools. School Environmental Inspection Report. 2005. Reports can be found at the BPS website at www. http://boston.k12.ma.us/
16. For the raw data, contact the Boston Public Schools Department.

Postscript

Since the *Who's Sick at School: Linking Poor School Conditions and Health Disparities for Boston's Children* report was released in 2006, MassCOSH and the BUAC have continued to successfully advocate for asthma-friendly schools and environmental policies in the BPSs to improve health and learning.

The coalition's approach includes working with the school staff unions, building parent leadership, and engagement in an active collaboration with the Boston Public Health Commission and Boston School department that has also linked this work with a broader "wellness" initiative. BUAC's advocacy and organizing approach has been adopted as a model in the formation of the Massachusetts Advocacy Action Partnership (MAAP) which completed a 5-year statewide asthma plan in May 2009 in conjunction with the Massachusetts Department of Public Health.

BUAC's Healthy Schools Committee continues to develop and evaluate its own advocacy action plan and meets quarterly with a city-wide Healthy Schools Taskforce with the school and health department. It has utilized community meetings, local media, Boston City Council ordinances and hearings to both pressure the city and school department to improve environmental management systems and to partner with them to pilot and adopt policies such as the replacement of conventional cleaners with green cleaners and a campaign to reduce clutter for better pest control. Compliance with the city ordinance to conduct twice annual environmental assessments, won through coalition pressure, have now been conducted for 6 years with some reductions in the percentage of schools with noted leaks, pests, and mold. The coalition continues to work with the school department to verify the accuracy of these inspections and foster accountability at the administrative levels for improving work-order systems, tracking asthma rates, and communicating with school staff and parents about best practices to reduce asthma triggers and improve air quality. Building on the success of implementing green cleaning in the Boston Schools, the City of Boston expanded upon that policy in July 2006 by requiring the use of green cleaners in all city buildings. The city has adopted green and healthy building standards that also apply to major school renovation projects.

As we face the current budget crisis in 2009-2010, the coalition has focused on improvements that will not require new funding. We have worked closely with the custodial union to make sure that there are no cuts in staffing levels for regular cleaning and maintenance. The coalition is pressing for the expansion of the software system that would capture all relevant information about the condition of a Boston school building.

BUAC believes that it will enable schools to better manage day-to-day maintenance and long-term capital repairs or renovations and to make school facility information more accessible to the community during the school budget process. At the same time, BUAC recognizes that the city has limited financial resources and joins with MassCOSH and healthy school advocates statewide to assess opportunities to receive federal stimulus or other funds for green school and energy efficiency projects that can be prioritized for communities most in need.

June 2012 Update on *Who's Sick at School* Report

Tolle Graham, Jean Zotter, and Marlene Camacho

Since the report *Who's Sick at School: Linking Poor School Conditions and Health Disparities for Boston's Children* was released in 2006, MassCOSH and the Boston Urban Asthma Coalition (now the Boston Healthy Homes and Schools Collaborative (BHHSC)) have continued to advocate successfully for asthma-friendly schools and environmental policies in the Boston Public Schools to improve health and learning. The coalition approach includes working with the school staff unions, building parent leadership, and engagement in an active collaboration with the Boston Public Health Commission and Boston School Department, which has also linked this work with a broader "wellness" initiative.

BHHSC's advocacy and organizing approach has been adopted as a model in the formation of the Massachusetts Advocacy Action Partnership (MAAP), which completed a five-year statewide asthma plan in May 2009 in conjunction with the Massachusetts Department of Public Health. This model was expanded to other communities with funding support from the U.S. Environmental Protection Agency and the Massachusetts Department of Public Health. The Greater Brockton Asthma Coalition and the Pioneer Valley Asthma Coalition have had success using this model in improving the school environments in their communities.

BHHSC's Healthy Schools Committee continues to develop and evaluate its own advocacy action plan and meets quarterly with a city-wide Healthy Schools Taskforce with the school and health department. It has utilized community meetings, local media, Boston City Council ordinances and hearings to both pressure the city and school department to improve environmental management systems and to partner with them to pilot and adopt policies such as the replacement of conventional cleaners with green cleaners and a campaign to reduce clutter for better pest control. Compliance with the City Ordinance to conduct twice-annual environmental assessments, won through coalition pressure, has now been the norm for seven years, with some reductions in the percentage of schools with noted leaks, pests, and mold. The coalition continues to work with the school department to verify the accuracy of these inspections and foster accountability at the administrative levels for improving work order systems, tracking asthma rates, and communicating with school staff and parents about best practices to reduce asthma triggers and improve air quality. Building on the success of implementing green cleaning in the Boston Schools, the City of Boston expanded upon that policy in July 2006, requiring the use of green cleaners in all city buildings. The City has adopted green and healthy building standards and in 2011 acquired a three-year funded position for a "Green Fellow" from the U.S. Green Building Council (USGBC).

As we have faced an increasing budget crisis over the last few years, the coalition has focused on improvements that will not require new funding. We have worked closely with the custodial union to make sure that there are no cuts in staffing levels for regular cleaning and maintenance and have targeted best practices for implementing integrated pest management with all school staff to reduce pests and clutter. The coalition is pressing for the expansion of the software system used in other city departments that would capture all relevant information about the condition of a Boston School building. BHHSC believes that this will enable schools to better manage day-to-day maintenance and long-term capital repairs or renovations and to make school facility information more accessible to the community during the school budget process.

CHAPTER 3

Failing Our Children: Lead in U.S. School Drinking Water*

Yanna Lambrinidou, Simoni Triantafyllidou, and Marc Edwards

Lead is the most prevalent toxicant in U.S. school drinking water. Yet for the vast majority of schools, federal regulation for testing taps and remediating contamination is voluntary. Using school case studies, this paper discusses the regulatory vacuum that leaves children unprotected from potential exposure to very high lead doses through consumption of school water. Controlling lead hazards from water fountains, coolers, and other drinking water outlets in schools requires improved sampling protocols that can capture the inherent variability of lead release from plumbing and measure both the particulate and dissolved lead present in water. There is a need to reevaluate the potential public health implications of lead-contaminated drinking water in schools. Accounting for this misunderstood and largely overlooked exposure source is necessary to better understand and address childhood lead poisoning in the United States.

In September 2007, children at Woodlake Avenue Elementary School in the Los Angeles suburb of Woodland Hills informed their parents that teachers had advised them not to drink the water from the school's fountains. Alarmed by the warning, the father of a first-grader requested that the Los Angeles Unified School District (LAUSD) test the school's water outlets immediately for hazardous contaminants. After several weeks of inaction, LAUSD sampled Woodlake's taps and returned in November to announce the results. One fountain dispensed water containing more than five times the concentration of lead

*A version of this chapter was originally published in the peer-reviewed journal *New Solutions* in 2010. Although the school cases featured have been investigated up to 2009, the chapter continues to reflect the status and policy of lead in U.S. school drinking water.

considered acceptable for school drinking water by the Environmental Protection Agency (EPA) (≤ 20 parts per billion (ppb)) and was shut off [1]. LAUSD promised school-wide replacement of drinking water fountains and lead-bearing plumbing materials at Woodlake but several weeks later had not begun the work. Troubled by the inertia, in January 2008 the father contacted a local television news station, which launched a district-wide investigation of lead in drinking water in the LAUSD. In March, undercover reporters collected samples from 30 schools and discovered that nine had at least one drinking water outlet that tested high for lead (> 20 ppb). Among those outlets was the very fountain at Woodlake that had been found to dispense elevated levels in the fall and was shut off. Four months after its initial sampling, the reporters found this fountain back in service, without evidence that it had undergone repairs [2].

In its exchanges with parents, LAUSD consistently asserted that the problem at Woodlake was a new discovery. When pressed by the news station, however, district officials admitted that tests eight years earlier had revealed elevated lead concentrations in water at several district schools, including Woodlake. In fact, according to an internal district report, widespread problems with lead in drinking water in the LAUSD schools had first been detected in 1988. To address the contamination, in 1990 LAUSD established a flushing policy, which required running the water for 30 seconds at every fountain in every school at the beginning of each school day [3, 4]. LAUSD's flushing program was based on a 1989 EPA guidance that listed flushing as an "interim measure" for reducing lead in water that can accumulate in school outlets when not in use [5].

To assess how LAUSD's policy was implemented at Woodlake and other district schools, the undercover reporters expanded their investigation to the daily routines of school custodians. They noted persistent failures to flush drinking water outlets as well as falsification of "flushing logs," indicating that flushing had occurred when it had not. In April 2008, the news station informed LAUSD about its findings. Days later, the district's superintendent held a little-announced press conference in which he attributed the contamination to possible employee non-compliance with the flushing policy. He declared that although negligent staff would be held accountable, failure of LAUSD to flush taps "did not put any students in jeopardy" [1]. When asked why the district had not addressed the contamination sooner, the superintendent replied that in a democracy school officials depended on the public to raise problems of this nature [6].

The press conference, held seven months after the Woodlake father's original plea for action, was the district's first official acknowledgement of persistent lead-in-water problems at LAUSD [7]. LAUSD assured the public that it had begun sampling randomly selected drinking water fountains and was planning to remediate all those that exceeded EPA's standard. It stressed that the district did not have the estimated $300 million needed to replace all lead-bearing plumbing at the schools, but that it was committed to fixing the worst problems. Based on the limited number of test results available at the time, LAUSD's superintendent asserted that the district's school water was "safe." "There is no reason for hysteria here," he stated [7]. The Woodlake father felt differently. "I am very concerned about [the contamination]," he said in a televised news interview, "because we don't even know really the long-term effects of this, or even the short-term effects, and we don't know how long the kids have been exposed to this" [8].

In May 2008, LAUSD began a multi-media and multi-language outreach effort to allay parent fears. As part of this campaign, it brought to Woodlake Elementary a pediatric toxicologist from the Los Angeles County Department of Public Health to educate parents about the potential health impact of the contamination. The County official declared that unless students had been chewing on lead paint chips there was little to worry about, and that in fact ordinary foods and drinks contained more lead than the school's water. "If you eat one Brussels sprout, you are going to get far more lead from that one Brussels sprout than you will get from weeks of drinking water here," he said. "I guarantee you, that if you tested the milk, the soda, the juice, the water that your child gets in your own home, it dwarfs the lead that your child is getting exposed to here" [9]. Taking up the toxicologist's challenge, the news station commissioned testing of all the cited food and beverage items and revealed undetectable levels of lead in every case [9].

As promised, LAUSD installed copper pipes and new water fountains at Woodlake. It also invested extensive resources to determine the extent of the contamination district-wide. In November 2008, it initiated comprehensive sampling of all drinking water outlets in all 735 schools at a cost of $1.5 million. Five months and more than 66,000 tests later, LAUSD announced plans to turn off indefinitely and replace more than 2,000 fountains and faucets due to high levels of lead [10]. An internal presentation for the district's Human Relations Committee and the School Safety, Student Health and Human Services Committee specified that these outlets exceeded the EPA standard for school taps in *both* first- and second-draw samples [11]. Some samples were tens and hundreds of times the EPA standard. In at least one of the samples, lead was measured at a level sufficient to classify the drinking water as "hazardous waste" (> 5,000 ppb lead) [12]. Approximately 7,000 additional outlets tested high for lead only in first-draw samples. LAUSD kept these outlets in service and committed to remediating them through daily flushing. All in all, contaminated taps were identified in 92 percent of the district's schools during 2008-2009 [13].

THE NATIONAL SCOPE OF THE PROBLEM

The LAUSD story typifies how many K-12 schools around the nation manage lead-in-water problems and highlights a systemic neglect of an environmental health hazard. School case studies reveal a pattern of incomplete understanding about how lead-bearing plumbing materials can release lead into water and what health risks contaminated water can pose. This pattern often leads to:

1. inertia vis-à-vis the identification and remediation of contamination;
2. reactive and suboptimal water testing programs in response to pressure from parents, teachers, and individuals outside the school community;
3. resistance to information-sharing concerning testing protocols, analytical methods, test results, and solutions;
4. delays in announcing contamination problems and avoidance of discussions about their potential health effects;
5. adoption of remedial measures that are logistically and/or financially burdensome, rooted in outdated scientific understandings of lead corrosion, or implemented inappropriately, incompletely, and without proof of effectiveness;
6. delivery of reassuring public health messages prematurely and/or without firm grounding in scientific facts; and
7. a sense of confidence and certainty when unknowns abound.

As a result, the unnecessary exposure of children to lead in school drinking water is often prolonged before protective action is taken—if ever.

In September 2009, the Associated Press (AP) released a nationwide investigation showing that lead-contaminated drinking water affects schools in at least 27 states [14]. AP's analysis was based on data from EPA, which are limited to the 8 to 11 percent of the country's 132,500 schools required by law to sample their taps for hazardous contaminants and to report results to state authorities. These schools are categorized as regularly providing drinking water to at least 25 individuals a day and using their own water source (e.g., private well) or treating or selling their water, and are thus regulated as "public water systems" [15]. The rest of the nation's schools, which receive their water from local utilities, are not subject to federal regulation, and EPA has no direct oversight responsibility for the quality of the drinking water they provide. Some of these schools have tested their water voluntarily and, in some cases, have discovered serious lead contamination. Our research shows that when this category of schools is taken into account, the number of states documented as affected by lead-contaminated school drinking water increases to at least 39 (including the District of Columbia). There is no scientific or practical reason to believe that the problem does not extend to schools in all 50 states.

A 2006 analysis by the U.S. Government Accountability Office (GAO) revealed that few states have developed comprehensive testing and remediation programs for lead in school drinking water, and about half the states have developed no programs at all [16]. Because many schools do not test for lead in drinking water, national data on the problem are limited. As a result, the true extent to which children in the United States are exposed to lead from school taps is unknown. What is evident, however, is that few schools have adopted measures to prevent such exposures. State and local officials correctly attribute this omission to the regulatory vacuum that leaves the vast majority of schools with no mandatory requirements for testing, unclear guidance on remediation, and little to no information about the potential health risks of lead at the tap.

Although the conventional wisdom is that lead in school drinking water poses little health risk, substantive gaps in policymakers' understanding of lead corrosion, proper water testing methods, and the research on childhood lead poisoning from contaminated water may have caused the impact of exposure to be underestimated.

WHO REGULATES LEAD IN U.S. SCHOOL DRINKING WATER?

For the approximately 90 percent of U.S. schools that receive their water from local utilities, no local, state, or federal entity is required to ensure that water lead levels are acceptably low (Table 1). Although some states and regional EPA offices have, at their discretion, encouraged and even facilitated sampling at school taps, water lead levels at the majority of the nation's schools are not monitored or remediated routinely, if ever. Thus, responsibility for addressing potential problems is effectively delegated to parents, teachers, and individuals outside the school community who are usually unsuspecting of lead-in-water contamination, unaware of the health risks it might pose, unable to implement testing and remediation programs, and trusting that if there were a significant environmental hazard at school it would be controlled effectively and expediently by experts.

Comprehensive federal regulation of drinking water safety in the United States was introduced in 1974. It was spurred by several influential studies that reported widespread problems with the safety of the nation's drinking water [17, 18]. To "assure that water supply systems serving the public [met] minimum national standards for protection of public health" [19], Congress passed the Safe Drinking Water Act (SDWA) of 1974. The SDWA authorized EPA to establish enforceable Maximum Contaminant Levels (MCLs) for all substances in drinking water with known or suspected adverse effects on human health. These minimum water quality requirements were to apply to every public water system in the country, including schools and child-care facilities regulated as public water systems. Federal and state agencies, as well as local water supply systems, were to take a central role in implementing the new law.

The EPA's National Interim Primary Drinking Water Regulations of 1975 kept 50 ppb, the standard set by the U.S. Public Health Service (PHS) in 1962, as the maximum allowable concentration of lead in drinking water [20]. The EPA's requirement, like that of the PHS, applied at the point where the water enters the distribution system rather than at consumer taps. It was, therefore,

Table 1. U.S. School Testing and Remediation Requirements for Lead in Water

	Schools regulated as public water systems	Schools not regulated as public water systems
Characteristics	Schools regularly provide water to an average of at least 25 individuals a day *and* have their own water source, or treat their water, or sell their water.	Schools receive drinking water from a public water system that is owned by a city, town, or other entity and neither treat nor sell this water.
Prevalence	8-11% of schools	89-92% of schools
Pertinent regulation	Federally mandated LCR: Under the SDWA's LCR, schools are *required* to sample water for lead regularly, remediate, and report results to the public as well as to state/federal authorities.	Voluntary LCCA: No federal law requires sampling for lead in water, although a small number of public water utilities include very limited school sampling in their LCR compliance monitoring. The implementation and enforcement of the SDWA's LCCA is at each state's discretion. Under the LCCA, EPA provides schools with guidance for a *voluntary* lead-in-water reduction program. Several states (and regional EPA offices) have taken an active role in ensuring some school sampling and remediation as well as educating school communities about lead at the tap.

Testing requirements	Testing *must* occur at a fixed number of taps (5-60, depending on the size of the population served) every 6 months, unless the school qualifies for reduced monitoring.	Under the LCCA, EPA *recommends* that, at a minimum, every school water outlet regularly used for drinking and cooking is sampled for lead. There are no requirements for frequency of sampling.
"Failure criterion" triggering remediation	Over 10% of 1-L samples exceed 16 ppb lead (LCR action level federally mandated).	Over 20 ppb lead in any 250 mL first-draw water sample (LCCA recommendation).
Remediation requirements	Under the LCR, remediation *requirements* include corrosion control optimization, public education, and lead service line replacement.	Under the LCCA, EPA *recommends* that any water outlet that fails the 20 ppb criterion be taken out of service and/or remediated.
Reporting requirements to state or federal agency with primary over enforcement of the SDWA	Schools serving fewer than 3,300 individuals are *required* to report a 90th percentile lead value only when over 10% of 1-L samples exceed 15 ppb lead. Larger school communities are *required* to report a 90th percentile lead value at every sampling round.	Under the LCCA, EPA *recommends* that schools make all test results available to the public, but it does not specifically require reporting to state or federal agencies.

guaranteed to miss the main source of the problem: namely, leaching of lead from lead service lines, lead solder, and indoor plumbing materials [21]. Hence, the original SDWA made it easy for public water systems to meet the 50 ppb MCL, even if the water provided by those systems dispensed hazardous levels of lead at drinking water outlets [22]. In 1977, the National Academy of Sciences acknowledged that "the present limit of 50 μg/liter may not, in view of other sources of environmental exposure, provide a sufficient margin of safety, particularly for fetuses and young growing children" and recommended that the allowable concentration of lead in drinking water be lowered [23].

Increasing recognition that lead can leach from plumbing materials *after* the water has left the treatment plant, and an EPA estimate that "as many as 250,000 children [had] suffered measurable IQ losses as the result of drinking lead-contaminated water" [24], led to the passage of three important federal statutes, which expanded the SDWA's regulatory reach to the tap [25].

The Lead Ban of 1986

This provision outlawed the new installation of solder and flux containing more than 0.2 percent lead and the use of pipes and pipe fittings containing more than 8 percent lead in all public water systems and in all buildings supplying drinking water for human consumption. Plumbing materials meeting these specifications were considered "lead-free" [26].

The Lead Contamination and Control Act (LCCA) of 1988

New tests by EPA, which showed that drinking-water coolers often contained lead solder or lead-lined tanks, prompted Congress to add a new provision to the SDWA. Based on concerns that water coolers were commonplace in schools, the LCCA characterized all refrigerated water fountains that did not meet EPA's definition of "lead-free" as "imminently hazardous consumer products" [27]. It banned their manufacture for, and sale in, interstate commerce and required their manufacturers and importers to repair, replace, or recall them. The LCCA also mandated that EPA issue guidance instructing all schools on how to identify and remediate lead-contaminated drinking water. It required states to disseminate this guidance and develop programs that would help school officials implement testing and remediation procedures and inform parents, teachers, and other employees about test results [5]. The LCCA did not make testing or remediation in schools mandatory, however.

In January 1989, EPA issued the first federal guidance on assessing and remediating lead in school drinking water. With this guidance, the agency announced a new lead-in-water standard for schools and urged the immediate disuse and remediation of taps that did not meet it. "In light of recent studies which reveal that even low levels of lead in drinking water can have subtle adverse effects on children," stated the guidance, "EPA recommends that action be taken to limit exposure or reduce lead in water whenever lead levels exceed 20 ppb" [5]. The new standard, applied to a 250-milliliter (mL) sample taken immediately after overnight stagnation and prior to any flushing, was based neither on health risk nor on expected health outcomes. It was merely a trigger for remedial action. The sampling protocol prescribed was designed to identify water outlets dispensing high lead and pinpoint the sources of identified contamination.

The passage of the LCCA, together with the dissemination of EPA's guidance, prompted many schools to test for lead in drinking water. However, an EPA audit in 1990 revealed that state adoption and enforcement of the regulation was often weak or even nonexistent [28]. Many schools had not repaired or removed lead-tainted coolers, had used sampling protocols other than the one recommended by EPA, had carried out very limited or inappropriate sampling, or had failed to conduct water testing at all. This overall anemic reaction to the LCCA on the state level mirrored EPA's own stance toward its new provision. The following is a typical response from a state official to an EPA questionnaire about how states were implementing the LCCA:

> Quite frankly, I'm disappointed at EPA's inconsistency and lack of leadership or direction with regard to this Act. On June 15, 1989, I received from EPA a letter which states "EPA has no official expectations of States in implementing the LCCA." If the Agency has "no expectations," then what is the purpose of the questionnaire? . . . Why must the state be placed in a position of defending our lack of attention to a non-funded federal program with no official expectations? [28].

At the same time, EPA auditors reported that harmful concentrations of lead continued to flow out of school water outlets, and that both EPA and states needed to be more aggressive in protecting children from unnecessary exposure to lead at the tap [29]. Six years later, a court ruling in the case of *ACORN v. Edwards*, 81 F.3d 1387 (5th Cir. 1996) held that provisions in the section of the LCCA compelling states to enact and enforce a federal regulatory program without having the option to decline were unconstitutional. This decision did not prohibit states from developing lead-in-water initiatives, but it also did not encourage a "more aggressive" approach to lead contamination at school taps, as had been recommended by EPA auditors. According to the GAO, state efforts in this regard were limited [16]. Moreover, they were never funded.

The EPA's most recent revision of its guidance to schools was published in 2006. Titled "3Ts for Reducing Lead in Drinking Water in Schools," it is based on the principle that controlling lead in school drinking water requires:

- proper *training* of school officials on the nature of lead at the tap, appropriate testing methods, and health risks of exposure;
- proper *testing* of drinking water; and

- proper *telling* to school communities about sampling programs, test results, remedial actions, and potential health effects.

The comprehensive, if not daunting, 100-page document opens with a prominently featured disclaimer: "This manual contains recommendations on how to address lead in school drinking water systems; these are suggestions only and are not requirements" [30].

The Lead and Copper Rule (LCR) of 1991

With the goal of reducing exposure to lead-tainted drinking water nationwide, in 1991 the EPA promulgated the first federal law regulating lead at the tap in communities served by public water systems through corrosion control and routine water monitoring. The LCR replaced the 1962 PHS lead-in-water standard of 50 ppb at the distribution system entry point with a maximum contaminant level *goal* (MCLG) of zero at the tap. As an MCLG, this standard was not enforceable, but represented the optimal lead-in-water level below which there was "no known or expected risk to health" [31]. The LCR also introduced a "lead action level" of 15 ppb in a one-liter (1-L) sample for the purpose of assessing corrosion control on a community-wide scale (the LCCA guideline of 20 ppb in a 250 mL sample corresponds to approximately 12 ppb in a 1-L sample) [32]. Like the school water standard, the LCR's lead action level was not health-based. It was derived from an estimation of lead concentrations considered at the time economically and technologically feasible to assess. Under the LCR, every public water system was required to evaluate regularly the presence and severity of lead contamination in the communities it served by identifying worst-case lead-in-water levels at drinking water taps in high-risk homes (e.g., with lead service lines or lead solder). If more than 10 percent of samples exceeded 15 ppb, public water systems were to intensify water quality monitoring, optimize corrosion control, issue public notification and education materials, and in some cases monitor and replace lead service lines [32]. Schools regulated as public water systems were also required to comply with the LCR.

Since 1991, significant progress has been made in monitoring lead-in-water levels in cities and towns across the country and at 8 to 11 percent of U.S. schools. The LCR, however, allows up to 10 percent of sampled taps to dispense any amount of lead without triggering remediation and public notification requirements. This means that, unless the contamination in a community or school is extensive, it can legally be left unaddressed. In May 2004, former U.S. Senators Jim Jeffords (I-VT) and Paul Sarbanes (D-MD), as well as U.S. Delegate Eleanor Holmes Norton (D-DC) and U.S. Representative Henry Waxman (D-CA), introduced the Lead-Free Drinking Water Act of 2005 [33, 34]. As a proposed amendment to the SDWA, this bill directed EPA to promulgate regulations requiring every state to develop a program under which schools licensed by the state would conduct annual testing for lead in drinking water and remediate any problems that were identified. The bill authorized EPA to provide funding to each state in order to assist schools with the costs of the program. The bill did not pass. It was reintroduced in 2005 and again in 2007, but it never became law [35-37].

WHY LEAD IN SCHOOL DRINKING WATER IS A HEALTH CONCERN

Lead is widely recognized as one of the most pervasive and serious environmental health threats in the United States, especially for children. In the last few decades, dramatic progress has been made to reduce lead exposure from gasoline, paint, dust, food and drink cans, and drinking water [38-40]. Despite these improvements, however, clinical evidence has recently demonstrated adverse health impacts at blood lead levels (BLLs) below the Centers for Disease Control and Prevention's (CDC's) 10 micrograms per deciliter (μg/dL) "level of concern" [41-44]. In light of the fact that decreased IQ and cognition have been linked to BLLs as low as 3 μg/dL, in May 2012 CDC replaced the federal "level of concern" with a "reference value" of 5 μg/dL, reinforcing the notion that there is no safe level of lead exposure [41-45]. Prior to that change, and for over two decades, BLLs above 10 μg/dL were referred to as "elevated blood lead levels" (EBLLs) or as "lead poisoning" in some jurisdictions. In 2000, the federal government adopted as one of its national health objectives the elimination of EBLLs in U.S. children by 2010 [46]. There was near universal acknowledgment from public health experts that this goal would not be met for many more years, and the date target was eventually abandoned [47].

The harmful health effects from lead exposure through drinking water have been formally recognized since the 1850s when such exposure was linked to high infant mortality, spontaneous abortion, neurological diseases, and digestive problems. Historian Werner Troesken suggested that use of lead pipes in major cities produced one of the most serious environmental health disasters in U.S. history [48]. Millions of lead pipes are still present in service lines in front of buildings throughout the United States, and lead-bearing plumbing materials can still cause very serious lead contamination of water (above 100 ppb lead), even in new construction [49]. Although health effects and exposure pathways vary dramatically from person to person, in part due to differences in individual water and food consumption patterns, lifestyles, and genetic risk factors [50, 51], lead exposure from drinking water is currently believed to account for 10 to 20 percent of total lead exposure on average in the general population, and for 40 to 60 percent of total lead exposure on average in infants dependent on reconstituted formula [52].

Our recent research has demonstrated that the potential contribution of lead in water to blood lead in children may have been underestimated. First, we discovered that the standard EPA methods used to assess the concentration of lead in drinking water can sometimes miss up to 99 percent of the lead that is actually present [53, 54]. Second, we demonstrated that in several recent cases of childhood lead poisoning from water, the affected children were not directly drinking the contaminated water. Rather, they were exposed from pasta and other foods that had been cooked in that water [53, 54]. Prior research did not consider the likelihood that lead in water could concentrate in food, or that food preparation could serve as a major pathway of lead exposure due to the large volume of water that is often used for cooking [53, 54]. Finally, we determined that in at least one U.S. city (Washington, DC), in 2000-2007 the incidence of blood lead poisoning for children less than 1.3 years of age was directly correlated with the levels of lead in their drinking water [55].

Children in many major cities are routinely screened for EBLLs, typically around age 1 and 2 years, if at all. In two recent cases of severe lead poisoning in school-aged children through accidental ingestion of lead-containing particles in jewelry, the affected children were initially misdiagnosed at the emergency room with symptoms of a viral infection and sent home [56, 57]. In one case, medical personnel finally noted via X-ray that lead was present in the child's stomach, but it was too late. The child went into respiratory arrest and died [57]. As a result of this incident, and because health problems resulting from consumption of lead in children's playthings often go undetected, decisive action was taken to protect school-aged children nationally from acute lead hazards (i.e., lead concentrations that if ingested even once can cause sudden and severe elevations in a child's BLL). In 2004, the U.S. Consumer Product Safety Commission (CPSC) recalled more than 150 million children's jewelry pieces, and the following year, after announcing that it was "aware of several cases in which children developed high blood lead levels after swallowing or repeatedly sucking on jewelry items," it established 175 micrograms (μg) of lead as a dose triggering acute health concerns [58]. This lead dose (175 μg is equivalent to 700 ppb in a 250 mL glass of water) was exceeded in drinking water samples collected at 10.3 percent of schools in Washington, DC, based on sampling conducted in 2007, even after 45 minutes of remedial flushing the night before.

If we, as a society, are concerned about a potential dose of 175 μg of lead from products such as toys and trinkets that are not intended for human consumption, we most certainly should be concerned about a similar dose of lead in drinking water. No prior studies of the hazards of lead in water at schools have explicitly considered acute health risks from ingestion of single glasses of water with worst-case levels of lead. Preliminary biokinetic modeling predicts that if a child were to consume a single 250-mL glass of water at the higher lead doses measured in schools (i.e., around 20,000 ppb lead), the child's blood lead would spike from 0 to over 50 μg/dL [55]. Levels of lead in the child's blood would remain above the CDC's 1991-2012 10 μg/dL "level of concern" for a period of weeks from a single exposure [55]. This acute elevation in BLLs can cause a variety of immediate common maladies, including abdominal discomfort, nausea, headaches, and gastrointestinal upset, as well as the long-term health concerns noted elsewhere [59].

Supporting our concern about the serious health risk posed by lead-contaminated water in schools, we uncovered a case of high BLLs in a Washington, DC, child attending an elementary school with lead-in-water problems during the city's historic 2001-2004 lead-in-water crisis. The highest lead-in-water measurement at this child's school was 7,300 ppb lead (i.e., 365 times the EPA lead standard for school taps). No other lead hazard was found in the child's home environment. We suspect that this case represents the tip of an iceberg of lead exposure risk. The vast majority of environmental risk assessments in Washington, DC, and nationally, whether conducted in 2001-2004 or at other times, do not include school water testing for lead, even when no lead hazards are identified in the home. Yet children's intermittent water consumption in schools—with periods of little or no water use on weekends, holidays and over summer break—regularly produces very long stagnation periods of water inside the piping. This water use pattern is considered "worst case" for causing release of hazardous levels of lead from the plumbing and contamination of the water supply [60-62]. Schoolchildren, especially those attending elementary school or day care centers, are much more vulnerable to adverse health effects from lead exposure than adults [61]. The combination of "worst-case" levels of lead in water and the presence of a vulnerable age group makes this issue of vital public health concern.

SOURCES OF LEAD IN SCHOOL WATER AND THE CHALLENGE OF ASSESSING CONTAMINATION

School buildings have intricate plumbing systems, sometimes very old, containing multiple potential sources of water contamination by lead. These include lead pipe, galvanized iron pipe, lead-containing solder joints, and system components made of lead-containing brass. In order to assess the public health risk from elevated lead in school drinking water, it is necessary first to determine the extent and severity of any contamination. This task can be challenging for several reasons. First, many schools and school districts are unaware that identifying and remediating lead in drinking water is solely their responsibility. Second, some schools and public water utilities sample school taps in a manner that hides lead problems. Third, even well-intentioned sampling efforts using standard protocols can inadvertently miss lead hazards. This is because of inherent variability in lead release from sample to sample, failure to capture lead particles in samples, and inadequate detection of lead particles when captured.

It has only recently been recognized that particulate lead can be the dominant form of lead in drinking water [63], and it is believed that lead particles are responsible for much of the lead in samples testing above 100 ppb lead in schools. Our own studies demonstrate that following the standard EPA sampling protocol can miss much of the particulate lead present in the water for the following reasons.

Under some circumstances, the likelihood that lead particles will be released into the water increases with flow rate. Yet EPA's school sampling instructions, which correctly promote replicating "typical water use patterns," recommend that bottles be filled with a "small," "pencil-sized" flow from the outlet [30]. This type of sampling procedure can artificially prevent the normally occurring release of lead particles and may not provide reliable information about lead levels in water consumed by children who use moderate or high flow rates to drink or fill water bottles from cafeteria, bathroom, and other school sinks.

Further, particulate lead can settle in or adhere to the plastic sampling containers, remaining undissolved even after acidification to pH < 2, as specified in EPA's standard procedures. This lead can be left behind in the bottle when the water is introduced to the analytical detector [53, 54]. As a result, the lead associated with lead particles can be missed. For example, a Washington, DC, water sample actually containing 508 ppb lead, measured as only 102 ppb using the standard EPA analytical protocol [64]. More recently, another sample, which actually contained more than 1,500 ppb lead, measured as only 3 ppb using procedures that are accepted by EPA. This latter sample would have provided false assurance that the water was "safe" based on EPA guidelines, when it was not. The presence of the higher concentration of lead was revealed only after vigorous mixing and stronger heated acid digestion steps were added to the protocol, so that the particulate lead was fully dissolved and quantified.

Finally, unlike the relatively steady presence of soluble lead in water, the mobilization of particulate lead from plumbing occurs sporadically. This means that repeated testing of some taps can produce multiple samples with low lead levels and a few samples with excessively high lead levels due to the release of lead particles. Current guidance, however, will "clear" a school tap as safe based on collection of a single sample below 20 ppb in a 250 mL sample, even if this tap periodically dispenses high levels of lead in particulate form.

As a result of these features of particulate lead contamination of water, even schools that strictly follow EPA's lead-in-water testing guidance are potentially missing significant lead hazards present in the water children routinely drink.

We have also demonstrated that in the more aggressive environment inside the human stomach (pH as low as 1.0, warm temperature, hydrochloric acid instead of nitric acid, mild agitation via churning), a large fraction of lead particles from brass, solder, lead pipe, and lead rust can dissolve and become bioavailable. Hence, lead in water that is missed by standard lab testing procedures can be absorbed once ingested [53, 54]. Our recent research on cases of childhood lead poisoning in Greenville, NC [65, 66], Washington, DC [67, 68], and Durham, NC [69], demonstrated that a key source of lead exposure was lead solder particles of about 1 to 100 micrometer diameter. It is our belief that the "worst case" lead levels detected in school water are often due to particulate lead, and that the reported lead concentrations in school samples are often lower than those to which U.S. children are actually exposed.

CASE STUDIES

The passage of the LCCA in 1988 heightened public awareness about potential health risks from lead-tainted water coolers and prompted many schools to test their drinking water for lead. Since then, numerous stories have appeared in the news media about problems with elevated lead in U.S. school drinking water. Although EPA has generally taken a back seat on the issue, two regional offices have assumed a more active role in helping schools protect children from hazardous levels of lead at school taps [70]. EPA Region I (serving New England) helped the Massachusetts Department of Environmental Protection to communicate with all schools in the state about lead in drinking water and supported efforts by Boston Public Schools to ensure that the water used to prepare school meals was not contaminated with lead. Similarly, EPA Region II (serving New Jersey, New York, Puerto Rico, the U.S. Virgin Islands, and eight tribal nations) developed a program that funds and provides technical support for lead-in-water sampling to schools in New York State and New Jersey. Early exemplary work was also done by EPA Region III (serving the mid-Atlantic region), which aggressively pursued lead-in-water problems at Philadelphia public schools [71].

Unfortunately, case studies across the country illustrate that most school communities remain unsupported in addressing lead-at-the tap contamination problems. The burden for complying with EPA guidance too frequently falls on concerned parents, teachers, and individuals outside the school community who sacrifice their personal time and resources to push school districts toward implementation of proactive testing and remediation programs. In case after case this burden is shouldered only after a prolonged exposure of children to high levels of lead in water, delayed parental notification about contamination problems, and questionable remedial measures, all of which can be expected to continue in the absence of a protective regulatory framework. The cases that follow are illustrative examples.

Los Angeles Unified School District

LAUSD first learned about problems with lead in school drinking water in 1988 [72]. It adopted flushing as a permanent solution but failed to ensure that the policy was implemented properly. It formally informed parents about the persistence of the contamination 20 years later, in response to pressure from a concerned parent and an undercover investigation by the media, but it coupled the news with false claims downplaying lead-in-water health risks and the potential health harm that may have already been done. For over two decades, LAUSD was controlling lead levels at approximately 9,000 taps via a single morning flush, which was not always carried out, and despite evidence that morning flushing can be unsuccessful at keeping lead levels low for the duration of the school day [73].

Washington, DC, Public Schools (DCPS)

DCPS was first made aware of lead-in-water problems in 1987. Initial tests showed some taps dispensing water with lead levels over 80 ppb. The school system characterized these results as "a matter of concern," but "not a health hazard" [74]. Seven years later, following a new round of testing, a television news station exposed that the district had failed to shut off several problem fountains, including one that had measured 1,520 ppb lead [75]. Following a January 2004 *Washington Post* story informing residents that excessive levels of lead had been flowing out of the city's taps for 2½ years, a third round of school samples was collected after first running the water for 10 minutes. Letting tap water run immediately before use is a well-known remedial measure for reducing lead when there are known contamination problems. Outcry about the invalid and misleading methodology led to limited re-testing, which revealed problems in 29 of 145 schools [76]. Later, however, it was discovered that, at the recommendation of the local water utility and EPA Region III, DCPS had conducted the re-testing with the use of still another sampling protocol that misses lead hazards. Specifically, water outlets were flushed for 10 minutes the night before sampling, and aerators, which can trap lead particles and release them slowly into the water, were removed. Despite the faulty methodology, some taps tested as high as 7,300 ppb. DCPS officials testified under oath that every problem tap would be remediated, but when questioned years later school officials revealed that no corrective action had been taken.

In 2006, lead-in-water elevations revealed in a new sampling round were not shared with the public until we obtained the results through a Freedom of Information Act request and forwarded them to the Washington, DC, City Council [77]. That testing round showed contamination in 12 of the 16 schools sampled. In one elementary school, 77 percent of the taps sampled measured above 20 ppb. Subsequent sampling at all schools in 2007 included running the water for 45-plus minutes on the night before sampling. The instruction was recommended by the local water utility and agreed to by EPA Region III, but when questioned by the press neither agency admitted responsibility for the sampling method employed [78]. Despite use of this unconventional protocol, results revealed contamination in 75 percent of DCPS schools. Fourteen schools had at least one tap dispensing water with lead levels above 700 ppb, the lead dose that CPSC classified in 2005 as an acute health concern for toys, trinkets, and consumer products. The highest lead-in-water measurement was 20,000 ppb. To address the contamination, DCPS installed lead filters at all drinking water fountains. In 2009, the district began a new testing round using the same 45-plus-minute flushing practice. Following complaints from the public, DCPS eventually promised to abandon the flawed instruction. It also agreed to allow parallel sampling by a team of independent scientists and community members. Testing has suggested that the filters are controlling lead-in-water levels effectively.

Baltimore City Public Schools (BCPS)

BCPS first became aware of lead-in-water contamination in 1992. Problem fountains were shut off, but later school administrators who were unaware of the issue reactivated them. In 2003, an investigation by a concerned father revealed that many of the fountains that had tested high 11 years earlier were still in operation. "Parents need to be alerted to the fact that their children are being placed in danger," he warned [79]. School officials admitted that many of the water outlets that had been disconnected in 1992-1993, "were somehow reactivated" in later years [80]. To eliminate the problem, BCPS announced the temporary closing of all water fountains at all schools and began to distribute bottled water. In 2004, the district turned back into service some fountains that tested below the EPA lead-in-water standard of 20 ppb and committed to flushing these outlets daily. Three years later, however, sampling at ten randomly selected schools by the city's Health Department revealed that 10 of 84 fountains, which had previously tested below 20 ppb, were again dispensing elevated levels of lead [81]. BCPS calculated that permanent use of bottled water would be cheaper than continued testing and potentially ineffective remediation. "Since our goal is 100 percent confidence," said the city's Commissioner of Health in November 2007, "the best approach is to switch to bottled drinking water" [82]. In 2003-2009, the district spent more than $2.5 million on bottled water [14].

Seattle Public Schools (SPS)

SPS first became aware of lead-in-water elevations in 1990. Most problem fountains and faucets were replaced, but testing two years later revealed persistent contamination in more than 40 schools [83]. A 1993 report recommended routine flushing of taps, the replacement of lead-bearing fountains, new pipes in four schools, and periodic sampling. Some water fountains were replaced, but the district did not implement a consistent program to address the contamination [84]. It also failed to officially notify the school community.

In December 2003, two fathers of students at Wedgwood Elementary School obtained SPS's 1993 report and discovered that four fountains at their children's school had tested high for lead a decade earlier. Out of concern about the orange color of the school's drinking water, they took samples from the very same fountains. Results revealed elevated lead levels in all samples, with the highest measurement at 200 ppb. "I think most citizens operate under the delusion that the safety of their children is being scrutinized by regulatory agencies in the schools," said one of the fathers. "It's quite the contrary" [85]. The EPA and the city's Health Department both denied responsibility.

SPS responded to the revelations by authorizing district-wide sampling and the delivery of bottled water to all schools built before 1997. Testing began in April 2004. Results showed that more than 70 percent of SPS schools had at least one water fountain with excessive levels of lead. In one school, 22 of the 24 fountains tested high [86]. In another, the fountain in the kindergarten and first grade class measured 1,600 ppb lead. The average lead level for that school's 27 fountains was 175 ppb [87]. At 19 schools, over half of the fountains had lead problems [83]. Twenty-six schools had fountains dispensing contaminated water even after flushing [88].

Local authorities contended that the contamination did not pose significant health risks, and a toxicologist hired by SPS opined that everything could be toxic in high enough doses, including pure water itself. In response to official statements that were perceived as downplaying the dangers of lead-contaminated water, one of the two fathers leading the campaign for safe water organized a public health forum that featured a nationally renowned expert in childhood lead poisoning and a leading water quality researcher. The two speakers offered a more sobering view of the health effects of lead in water, which convinced some Seattle School Board members to support the creation of a district-wide policy requiring regular and aggressive testing and remediation [89, 90].

SPS addressed the contamination by repairing or replacing all problem fountains and conducting limited replacement of school plumbing. The school board adopted its first drinking water policy in December 2004, which lowered the allowable lead level for school taps to 10 ppb and established requirements for water quality testing, remediation, and public notification every three years [91].

CONCLUSION

School case studies in Los Angeles, Washington DC, Baltimore, and Seattle highlight the potential exposure of sensitive populations to very high lead doses through consumption of contaminated drinking water. Lead levels greater than the EPA guideline of 20 ppb were measured at as many as 92 percent of taps in some schools, and some drinking water outlets released concentrations of lead sufficient to classify the water as "hazardous waste." Controlling lead hazards from drinking water at schools requires improved sampling protocols that can capture the inherent variability of lead release from plumbing and that can quantify both the particulate and dissolved lead present in water. Depending on the type of lead-in-water problems encountered, practical and concise remediation guidance is needed for school communities. Most importantly, the potential public health implications need to be re-evaluated. While the association between lead in water and lead in blood has been documented through decades of prior scientific research, the possible contribution of school drinking water lead to the body's total lead burden is not a current focus of public health policy. Accounting for this misunderstood and largely overlooked exposure source is necessary to better understand and address childhood lead poisoning in the United States.

ACKNOWLEDGMENTS

The authors acknowledge the financial support of the National Science Foundation (NSF) under grant CBET-0933246. Opinions and findings expressed herein are those of the authors and do not necessarily reflect the views of NSF. The authors also thank all the parents and government representatives who shared their experiences with us, as well as the high school student volunteers from the Washington International School and César Chávez Public Charter Schools for Public Policy in Washington DC, for their participation in water sampling at DC Public Schools in 2008 and 2009.

NOTES

1. J. Grover and M. Goldberg, "School Water Investigation," *KNBC* (Los Angeles), April 24, 2008, http://www.nbclosangeles.com/School_Water_Investigation.html (accessed May 15, 2012).
2. J. Grover, "Contaminated Water?" *KNBC* (Los Angeles), April 24, 2008, http://publichealth.lacounty.gov/lead/news/Joel%20Grover%20-%20Contaminated%20Water%20at%20Schools.pdf (accessed May 15, 2012).
3. E. Woo, "Lead Level Unsafe in 400 L.A. School Water Fountains," *Los Angeles Times,* November 22, 1988, http://articles.latimes.com/1988-11-22/local/me-424_1_drinking-fountains (accessed May 15, 2012).
4. P. Shenon, "Lead Going Unchecked in Schools," *Los Angeles Daily News,* November 1, 1990.
5. U.S. Environmental Protection Agency, "Lead in School's Drinking Water," pp. 20-21 (Report 570-9-89-001), January 1989.
6. S. Abram, "High Levels of Lead are Discovered in Valley School Drinking Fountain," *Los Angeles Daily News*, April 23, 2008.
7. S. Abram, "School Water Alarms Parents," *Los Angeles Daily News,* April 27, 2008.
8. S. Thoma, interview by Chris Schauble, *KNBC* (Los Angeles), 2008, http://www.nbclosangeles.com/news/health/LAUSD-Schools-Shut-Down-Faucets-Due-to-Lead-Levels.html (accessed May 15, 2012).
9. J. Grover and M. Goldberg, "School Water Investigation, Part 4: Is LAUSD Lying to Parents About Safety of Water in Schools?" *KNBC* (Los Angeles), May 14, 2008, http://www.nbclosangeles.com/news/Is_LAUSD_Lying_To_Parents_About_Safety_Of_Water_In_Schools__Los_Angeles.html (accessed May 15, 2012).
10. G. B. Sanchez, "Faucets Shut Off at Schools Due to High Lead Levels," *Los Angeles Daily News*, March 13, 2009.
11. Los Angeles Unified School District, "Lead in Water Mitigation Management," presentation, LAUSD School Safety, Student Health & Human Services Committee and Human Relations Committee, March 12, 2009, http://notebook.lausd.net/pls/ptl/docs/PAGE/CA_LAUSD/FLDR_ORGANIZATIONS/COMMITTEE_MAIN/COMMITTEE_SSHHS/COMMITTEE_SSHHS_AGENDA/2.%20UPDATE%20ON%20LEAD%20IN%20DRINKING%20WATER.PDF (accessed May 15, 2012).
12. Los Angeles Unified School District, Office of Environmental Health and Safety, "School Drinking Water Testing Results" (10th Street Elementary School, January 9, 2009), http://www.lausd-oehs.org/drinkingwater_results.asp (accessed May 15, 2012).

13. J. Grover and M. Goldberg, "LAUSD Testing Reveals Widespread Lead Contamination in Water," *KNBC* (Los Angeles), March 24, 2009, http://www.nbclosangeles.com/news/local-beat/LAUSD-Testing-Reveals-Widespread-Lead-Contamination-in-Water.html (accessed May 15, 2012).
14. G. Burke, "School Drinking Water Contains Toxins," *Associated Press*, September 25, 2009, http://seattletimes.nwsource.com/html/nationworld/2009942499_apustoxicwaterschools.html (accessed May 15, 2012).
15. U.S. Environmental Protection Agency, "Drinking Water in Schools & Child Care Facilities: Laws and Regulations," http://water.epa.gov/infrastructure/drinkingwater/schools/regulations.cfm (accessed May 15, 2012).
16. U.S. Government Accountability Office, "Drinking Water: EPA Should Strengthen Ongoing Efforts to Ensure that Consumers are Protected from Lead Contamination" (Report to Congressional Requesters, GAO 06-148), January 2006, http://www.gao.gov/new.items/d06148.pdf (accessed May 15, 2012).
17. W. E. Cox, "Evolution of the Safe Drinking Water Act: A Search for Effective Quality Assurance Strategies and Workable Concepts of Federalism," *William and Mary Environmental Law and Policy Review* 21 (1997): 69-164.
18. C. D. Larson, "Historical Development of the National Primary Drinking Water Regulations," in *Safe Drinking Water Act: Amendments, Regulations and Standards* (Chelsea, MI: Lewis Publishers, Inc., 1989), 3-15.
19. H.R. 93-1185, *Safe Drinking Water Act*, (1974): 1.
20. U.S. Environmental Protection Agency, "National Interim Primary Drinking Water Regulations" (EPA 570/9-76-003), 1976.
21. R. P. Maas et al., "Reducing Lead Exposure from Drinking Water: Recent History and Current Status," *Public Health Reports* 120 (2005): 316-321.
22. R. H. Gnaedinger, "Lead in School Drinking Water," *Journal of Environmental Health* 55, 6 (1993): 15-18.
23. National Academy of Sciences, Safe Drinking Water Committee, *Drinking Water and Health*, pp. 260-261 (Washington DC: National Academy of Sciences, 1977).
24. U.S. Department of Agriculture, *Selecting and Renovating an Old House: A Complete Guide*, p. 13 (Toronto, ON: General Publishing Company, Ltd., 2000).
25. M. Engel, "Fear of Lead in DC Water Spurs Requests for Tests," *Washington Post*, December 6, 1986.
26. U.S. Environmental Protection Agency, "The Lead Ban: Preventing the Use of Lead in Public Water Systems and Plumbing Used for Drinking Water" (EPA 57Q/9-89-BBB), August 1989.
27. U.S. Environmental Protection Agency, "History: Lead Contamination Control and Asbestos Information Acts of 1988" [press release], November 1, 1988, http://www.epa.gov/history/topics/sdwa/06.html (accessed September 22, 2009).
28. U.S. Environmental Protection Agency, "Report of Audit on the Lead in Drinking Water Program" (E1HWF9-03-0316-0100508), September 28, 1990.
29. P. Shenon, "Despite Law, Study Finds, Water in US Schools May Contain Lead," *New York Times*, November 1, 1990, http://www.nytimes.com/1990/11/01/us/despite-law-study-finds-water-in-us-schools-may-contain-lead.html (accessed May 15, 2012).
30. U.S. Environmental Protection Agency, "3Ts for Reducing Lead in Drinking Water in Schools: Revised Technical Guidance" (EPA 816-E-05-008), October 2006, http://www.epa.gov/ogwdw/schools/pdfs/lead/toolkit_leadschools_guide_3ts_leadschools.pdf (accessed May 15, 2012).

31. U.S. Environmental Protection Agency, "25 Years of the Safe Drinking Water Act: History and Trends" (EPA 816-R-99-007), December 1999, http://permanent.access.gpo.gov/websites/epagov/www.epa.gov/safewater/consumer/trendcvr.pdf (accessed May 15, 2012).
32. U.S. Environmental Protection Agency, "Lead and Copper Rule: A Quick Reference Guide" (EPA-816-F-04-009), March 2004, http://www.epa.gov/safewater/lcrmr/pdfs/qrg_lcmr_2004.pdf (accessed May 15, 2012).
33. S. 2377, Lead-Free Drinking Water Act of 2004, http://www.govtrack.us/congress/bill.xpd?bill=s108-2377 (accessed May 15, 2012).
34. H.R. 4268, Lead-Free Drinking Water Act of 2004, http://www.govtrack.us/congress/bill.xpd?bill=h108-4268 (accessed May 15, 2012).
35. S. 1328, Lead-Free Drinking Water Act of 2005, http://www.govtrack.us/congress/bill.xpd?bill=s109-1328 (accessed May 15, 2012).
36. H.R. 3178, Lead-Free Drinking Water Act of 2005, http://www.govtrack.us/congress/bill.xpd?bill=h109-3178 (accessed May 15, 2012).
37. H.R. 2076, Lead-Free Drinking Water Act of 2007, http://www.govtrack.us/congress/bill.xpd?bill=h110-2076 (accessed May 15, 2012).
38. P. J. Landrigan and A. C. Todd, "Lead Poisoning," *Western Journal of Medicine* 161 (1994): 153-159.
39. E. Millstone, *Lead and Public Health* (Washington, DC: Taylor & Francis, Inc. 1997).
40. R. A. Goyer, "Lead Toxicity: Current Concerns," *Environmental Health Perspectives* 100 (1993): 177-187.
41. R. L. Canfield et al., "Intellectual Impairment in Children with Blood Lead Concentrations Below 10 μg per Deciliter," *New England Journal of Medicine* 348 (2003): 1517-1526.
42. D. C. Bellinger and H. L. Needleman, "Intellectual Impairment and Blood Lead Levels," *New England Journal of Medicine* 349 (2000): 502.
43. B. P. Lanphear et al., "Cognitive Deficits Associated with Blood Lead Concentrations <10 microg/dL in US Children and Adolescents," *Public Health Reports* 115, 6 (2000): 521-529.
44. T. A. Jusko et al., "Blood Lead Concentrations < 10 μg/dL and Child Intelligence at 6 Years of Age," *Environmental Health Perspectives* 116, 2 (2008): 243-248.
45. Centers for Disease Control and Prevention (CDC). 2012. "CDC Response to Advisory Committee on Childhood Lead Poisoning Prevention Recommendations in "Low Level Lead Exposure Harms Children: A Renewed Call of Primary Prevention," http://www.cdc.gov/nceh/lead/ACCLPP/CDC_Response_Lead_Exposure_Recs.pdf (accessed May 22, 2012).
46. J. G. Schwemberger et al., "Blood Lead Levels—United States, 1999-2002," *Morbidity and Mortality Weekly Report*, 54, 20 (2005): 513-516, http://www.cdc.gov/mmwr/preview/mmwrhtml/mm5420a5.htm (accessed May 15, 2012).
47. HealthyPeople.gov. 2012. "Environmental Health," http://www.healthypeople.gov/2020/topicsobjectives2020/overview.aspx?topicid=12 (accessed May 22, 2012).
48. W. Troesken, *The Great Lead Water Pipe Disaster* (Cambridge: MIT Press, 2006).
49. C. Elfland and M. Edwards, "Managing and Resolving Lead Problems in Potable Water of New Construction" (Water Quality Technology Conference and Exhibition, American Water Works Association, Cincinnati, OH, November 16-20, 2008).

50. M. R. Hopkins et al., "Variants in Iron Metabolism Genes Predict Higher Blood Lead Levels in Young Children," *Environmental Health Perspectives* 116, 9 (2008): 1261-1266.
51. M. Shannon and J. W. Graef, "Lead Intoxication from Lead-Contaminated Water Used to Reconstitute Infant Formula," *Clinical Pediatrics* 28 (2009): 380-382.
52. U.S. Environmental Protection Agency, "Basic Information about Lead in Drinking Water," http://water.epa.gov/drink/contaminants/basicinformation/lead.cfm (accessed May 15, 2012).
53. S. Triantafyllidou, J. Parks, and M. Edwards, "Lead Particles in Potable Water," *Journal of the American Water Works Association,* 99, 6 (2007): 107-117.
54. S. Triantafyllidou, "Addressing and Assessing Lead Threats in Drinking Water: Non-Leaded Brass, Product Testing, Particulate Lead Occurrence and Effects of the Chloride to Sulfate Mass Ratio on Corrosion" (master's thesis, Virginia Tech, 2006).
55. M. Edwards, S. Triantafyllidou, and D. Best, "Elevated Blood Lead in Young Children Due to Lead-Contaminated Drinking Water: Washington, DC, 2001-2004," *Environmental Science and Technology* 43, 5 (2009): 1618-1623.
56. U.S. Centers for Disease Control and Prevention, "Brief Report: Lead Poisoning from Ingestion of a Toy Necklace–Oregon, 2003," *Morbidity and Mortality Weekly Report*, June 18, 2004, http://www.cdc.gov/mmwr/preview/mmwrhtml/mm5323a5.htm (accessed May 15, 2012).
57. U.S. Centers for Disease Control and Prevention, "Death of a Child After Ingestion of a Metallic Charm–Minnesota, 2006," *Morbidity and Mortality Weekly Report*, March 23, 2006, http://www.cdc.gov/mmwr/preview/mmwrhtml/mm55d323a1.htm (accessed May 15, 2012).
58. U.S. Consumer Product Safety Commission, Office of Information and Public Affairs, "CPSC Announces New Policy Addressing Lead in Children's Metal Jewelry," February 3, 2005, http://www.cpsc.gov/cpscpub/prerel/prhtml05/05097.html (accessed May 15, 2012).
59. S. Triantafyllidou and M. Edwards, Lead (Pb) in Tap Water and in Blood: Implications for Lead Exposure in the United States. *Critical Reviews in Environmental Science and Technology* 42, 13 (2012): 1297-1352.
60. R. M. Levin et al., "Lead Exposures in US Children, 2008: Implications for Prevention," *Environmental Health Perspectives* 116, 10 (2008): 1285-1293.
61. U.S. Environmental Protection Agency, "Control of Lead and Copper in Drinking Water" (EPA I 625®-93001), May 1993. http://www.epa.gov/nrmrl/pubs/625r93001/625r93001.pdf (accessed May 15, 2012).
62. S. Breese, "Factors Influencing the Rate of Lead Release in Domestic Plumbing Systems" (American Water Works Association Annual Conference and Exposition, Atlanta, GA, June 8-12, 2008).
63. L. S. McNeill and M. Edwards, "Importance of Pb and Cu Particulate Species for Corrosion Control," *ASCE Journal of Environmental Engineering* 130, 2 (2004): 136-144.
64. M. Edwards and A. Dudi, "Role of Chlorine and Chloramine in Corrosion of Lead-Bearing Plumbing Materials," *Journal of the American Water Works Association* 96, 10 (2004): 69-81.
65. J. Allegood, "Pitt Probes Boy's Lead Poisoning," *Raleigh News and Observer*, May 6, 2005.

66. S. T. Bachelor, "Area Family Copes with Lead Poisoning," *The Greenville Daily Reflector*, May 4, 2005.
67. L. Copeland, "Blood and Water: The Long Search for the Source of a Baby's Lead Poisoning," *Washington Post*, March 4, 2004.
68. R. Renner, "Mis-lead," *Environmental Science & Technology* 40, 14 (2006): 4333-4334.
69. R. Gronberg, "City Water Lead Levels Alarming Regulators," *The Herald-Sun*, June 26, 2006, http://www.herald-sun.com/durham/4-747728.html (accessed June 27, 2006).
70. U.S. Environmental Protection Agency, "Controlling Lead in Drinking Water for Schools and Day Care Facilities: A Summary of State Programs" (EPA-810-R-04-001), July 2004, http://www.epa.gov/safewater/lcrmr/pdfs/report_lcmr_schools summary.pdf (accessed May 15, 2012).
71. S. Fitzgerald, "District: Unsafe Lead Levels Found in 20 pct of Water Outlets," *Philadelphia Inquirer*, November 21, 2000.
72. E. Woo, "Lead Level Unsafe in 400 L.A. School Water Fountains," *Los Angeles Times*, November 22, 1988, http://articles.latimes.com/1988-11-22/local/me-424_1_drinking-fountains (accessed May 15, 2012).
73. E. A. Murphy, "Effectiveness of Flushing on Reducing Lead and Copper Levels in School Drinking Water," August 1993, http://ehp03.niehs.nih.gov/article/fetchArticle.action?articleURI=info%3Adoi%2F10.1289%2Fehp.93101240 (accessed May 9, 2012).
74. M. Fisher, "Excessive Lead Levels Found in Water at 10 DC Schools," *Washington Post*, December 24, 1987.
75. D. Cohn, "Leaded Water Still On in Some DC Schools," *Washington Post*, March 3, 1994.
76. A. Goldstein and J. Blum, "Tests Find Lead High at 29 DC Schools," *Washington Post*, April 30, 2004.
77. T. Labbe, "Tests Find Elevated Lead Levels at Five Schools, DC Council Told," *Washington Post*, February 15, 2007.
78. C. D. Leonnig, "Parents Demand New Tests of School Water," *Washington Post*, April 29, 2007.
79. Associated Press Newswires, "Fountains with Lead Remain in Schools," February 7, 2003.
80. Associated Press Online, "Baltimore Schools Close Water Fountains," February 7, 2003.
81. S. Neufeld, "All City Schools to Get Water Coolers," *Baltimore Sun*, November 8, 2007.
82. City of Baltimore, "Baltimore City Public Schools' CEO Announces System-Wide Shift to Bottled Drinking Water" [press release], November 7, 2007, http://www.baltimorecityschools.org/cms/lib/MD01001351/Centricity/Domain/87/PDF/Lead_in_Water110707.pdf (accessed May 15, 2012).
83. D. Bach, "Lead Dangers Stun Parents," *Seattle-Post Intelligencer*, July 2, 2004.
84. D. Bach, "Schools Will Bring in Water," *Seattle Post-Intelligencer*, December 18, 2004.
85. D. Bach, "From Concerned Parent to Crusader for Safe Water," *Seattle Post-Intelligencer*, August 18, 2004.

86. D. Bach, "Schools' Water Fails Lead Testing," *Seattle Post-Intelligencer*, April 30, 2004.
87. M. S. Cooper, "Get the Lead Out of Schools' Water," *Seattle Post-Intelligencer*, July 2, 2004.
88. Associated Press, "Tests Find High Lead Levels in Many School Water Fountains," July 2, 2004.
89. D. Bach, "Schools Can Cut Lead for Less, Expert Says," *Seattle Post-Intelligencer*, November 1, 2004.
90. S. Bhatt, "Report Says Lead Levels in Schools' Water Not Dire," *Seattle Times*, March 25, 2005.
91. Seattle Public Schools, "Drinking Water Quality Improvement Program: 2010-2011 Annual Report," http://www.seattleschools.org/modules/groups/homepagefiles/cms/1583136/File/Departmental%20Content/general%20counsel/Risk%20management/Drinking%20water%20quality/AnnualReport/AnnualReport_summary.pdf?sessionid=1d0fe12b422d4f58fc0cbddf8e55924c (accessed May 15, 2012).

CHAPTER 4

PCBs in School—Persistent Chemicals, Persistent Problems

Robert F. Herrick

The issue of polychlorinated biphenyls (PCB) exposures resulting from occupancy of PCB-contaminated buildings is not new, but the contribution of building materials to that contamination is largely unrecognized. A rapidly emerging base of evidence shows that PCBs can be widely found in caulking and paint in masonry buildings constructed or renovated from about 1950 to the late 1970s. These materials can cause extensive PCB contamination of the building interiors and surrounding soil, and people who teach, live, or attend school in these buildings can have elevated serum PCB levels. The potential risk associated with this source of PCB exposure is not known; however, it is worth noting that the specific PCB congeners found at high levels in the building environments, and in biological samples from the occupants, include some that are suspected of being potent neurotoxins. The U.S. Environmental Protection Agency (EPA) is moving to address this issue in schools; however, the costs of remediating contaminated buildings will pose a formidable obstacle to most school districts.

The story of PCB contamination in schools is unfinished. We know that PCBs got into schools in building materials such as window caulking and paints. Given the time that has passed since these buildings were constructed, and the number of buildings that have already been renovated and had the PCB materials removed, the precise significance of the risk that PCBs from these sources pose to children, teachers, and other occupants of the schools may never be known. Although the presence of PCB caulk and paint in these buildings causes PCB contamination of the building interiors and the soil around the buildings, and is a clear violation of the federal "Toxic Substances Control Act" (40 CFR

Part 761), the great majority of people who work, teach, or go to school in these buildings have no idea that they are being exposed to PCBs.

What is known is that PCBs can be present in buildings constructed or renovated from about the mid-1950s to the late 1970s, coinciding with a period of extensive school construction. Paints, the caulking material around window and door frames and in expansion joints and other building materials can contain very substantial amounts of PCB, sometimes in levels of hundreds of thousands of parts per million (ppm). For reference, the "Toxic Substances Control Act" (TSCA) prohibits material with PCB levels exceeding 50 ppm (40 CFR Part 761), and the U.S. Environmental Protection Agency considers this to be an "unauthorized use" of PCBs. It is also known that much of this material is at or near the end of its service life and is being replaced during building renovation projects, such as window replacements. In most cases, no precautions are taken to prevent the release of PCB-containing dust into the school environment while the old materials are scraped and ground out. This has resulted in extensive PCB contamination of building interiors and surrounding grounds. In other cases, the PCBs are being released from deteriorating caulk that is still in place but has weathered to the extent that the polymer is breaking down.

BACKGROUND

Indoor contamination with PCB is not new. It is very well documented that building environments can be contaminated as a result of transformer leaks, fires, and explosions. The EPA and states including California specifically addressed this source of PCB contamination, including some fact sheets targeted to schools [1, 2].

In the U.S., the possibility of indoor PCB contamination from building materials such as caulk and paint went largely unrecognized, despite the attention paid to PCB releases from transformers and other sources. Starting in the early 1990s, investigators in Germany, Sweden, and Finland reported the presence of PCB in building sealants (caulking) and demonstrated relationships between these PCBs and elevated PCB levels in indoor air and settled dust [3]. Other investigators confirmed these findings and found extensive contamination of soil around the foundations of buildings containing these materials [4-8]. The EPA stated in 1996 that "very little is known about contaminated caulking and grout, their specific applications and dissemination in the marketplace. Samples of caulking that have been contaminated with PCBs have been found in a setting previously used as a school at a maximum concentration of 310,000 ppm PCBs (Ref. 12)." This reference is to a U.S. Army Corps of Engineers report, "Final Site Investigation Report for Campbell, Lyle, Stone and Otis Memorial Schools, Bourne, MA" [9]. In covering this story, the *Boston Globe* (March 21, 1996) reported that the Corps of Engineers sampled caulking, ceiling tiles, and paint in an elementary school on the Massachusetts Military Reservation and found PCB levels up to 2,000 times greater than allowed under state rules [10].

In the late 1990s, investigations in Sweden and Germany found that teachers and students in schools containing PCB caulking were exposed to elevated levels of PCB in the indoor air. These exposures caused significantly elevated serum levels of specific PCB congeners that were released from building materials [11-14]. During a 2000 investigation conducted to address occupants' concerns about cancer and possible pesticide contamination in a university administration building [15, 16], PCB was detected in dust samples. The university closed the building, and subsequent testing revealed that gasket, foamboard insulation, and caulking material contained PCB in quantities up to 33,000 mg/kg (ppm). In the case of this university building, EPA (Region 1, Boston), mandated a clean-up program to remove the identified PCB-containing materials and clean the building to clearance criteria of 1 microgram per cubic meter ($\mu g/m^3$) in air, 10 micrograms/ 100 square centimeters in surface wipes, and 1 ppm in porous building components (brick and concrete blocks). This abatement was mandated under the EPA finding that the PCB concentrations in caulk and other building materials exceeded 50 ppm, which constituted "unauthorized use" of non-liquid PCB products. The total cost of the abatement of the building exceeded $2 million.

THE CURRENT SITUATION

In 2003, E. Priha (Finnish Institute of Occupational Health) made a presentation at the American Industrial Hygiene Conference and Exposition describing a national project to remove PCB caulk from buildings in Finland [17]. One finding of that national initiative was the estimate by Finnish authorities that 220 tons of PCB had been used in over 10,000 buildings. As of 2003, approximately 85% of that material had been replaced with non-PCB containing caulking material.

Was the situation in the U.S. similar to that reported in Finland? To seek an answer, researchers at the Harvard School of Public Health called upon the support of the International Union of Bricklayers and Allied Craft Workers and one of their retired members. We had collaborated with this retiree in The Center for Construction Research and Training-supported research on dust controls. He had specialized in pointing, cleaning and caulking (PCC) work, and he remembered installing PCB-containing caulk in buildings throughout New England. He collected small (~ 10 g) samples of caulking from the exterior of 24 buildings. At the time of the sampling (2003), some buildings had already undergone renovation and caulking appeared to have been replaced. In others, reconstruction projects were underway, and, in some others, the original caulking was still in place but was obviously deteriorated and peeling away from the building joints. Of the 24 buildings sampled, 13 contained caulking material in which detectable levels of PCBs were measured, and eight of these 13 contained caulking that exceeded the 50 ppm EPA removal criteria by a factor of nearly 1,000 (range, 70.5–36,200 ppm; mean, 15,645 ppm) [18]. The elevated PCB levels in caulking were found in schools, university buildings, and other public buildings (Table 1).

Table 1. Sampling Results from 24 Buildings in Greater Boston

Building type	PCB Content (ppm by mass)[a]
Government office, mixed use	35,600
Government office	25.2
Office building	Not detected[b]
Subsidized housing	Not detected
Subsidized housing	Not detected
Elderly housing	Not detected
Elderly housing	Not detected
University student housing	36,200
University dormitory	70.5
University dormitory	1.68
University classrooms and offices	26,400
Elementary school	7,740
Middle school	5,010
High school	5,970
High school	Not detected
High school	Not detected
Community college	19.3
Church offices	2.14
Synagogue	8,240
Hospital	Not detected
Hospital	Not detected
Museum	0.56
Hotel	Not detected
Police station	Not detected

[a]All samples, except for the sample from the governmental office/mixed use building, were identified as Aroclor 1254. This sample was identified as Aroclor 1260.

[b]Samples reported as "Not detected" contained PCB at less than the reporting limit, which ranged from 114-455 μg/kg (0.114-0.455 ppm).

This finding might have remained a scientific curiosity were it not for a concerned parent in Yorktown Heights, New York. Dr. Daniel Lefkowitz read the results of the sampling in Boston and wondered about his son's school which was built in 1969. Its windows had been replaced in 2003. He was curious to find out whether the caulking that had been removed in the window replacement contained PCBs, so he called the EPA Region 2. They advised him to look for a piece of caulking on the ground and send it to a lab for testing. He found a piece, had it tested (at his own expense), and got the result that the caulking contained 38,000 ppm PCB, 760 times the EPA's allowable limit.

Dr. Lefkowitz notified the Westchester County Department of Health of his finding, and they ordered the school to remove any remaining pieces of caulk on the ground. They refused Lefkowitz's request that the soil around the school be tested, so again he collected a sample and paid for the analysis himself. The soil sample came back with elevated levels of PCB above the New York State 1 ppm clean-up requirement. The Westchester Department of Health did its own soil testing and confirmed Lefkowitz's result of soil contamination, finding levels as high as 40 ppm (see Figure 1).

They ordered the school to fence off all of the contaminated areas and removed nearly 600 cubic yards of contaminated soil. The total cost of decontaminating the school was approximately $300,000, although the PCB caulking remaining in building expansion joints and around doors, etc. was encapsulated in paint, and not removed until 2007.

Lefkowitz's findings and concerns were met with some skepticism, but he persisted, and created a website www.pcbinschools.org to disseminate information on PCB contamination in schools. The Westchester County government sought the advice of the EPA, and in response to a letter from Michael Kaplowitz, Chairman of Budget and Appropriations Committee of the Westchester County Board of Legislators, Kenneth S. Stoller, the Chief of Pesticides and Toxic Substances Branch, EPA Region 2 stated:

> *"The use of PCBs in caulking and sealant materials has never been authorized by the Environmental Protection Agency. In general, the placement of such materials pre-dates the enactment of the Toxic Substances Control Act and its use today is not authorized. Therefore, the prospect of authorizing the continued use of this material in residential settings, or where children could be exposed, is extremely unlikely. Because it is illegal, and the potential for exposure may be significant, PCB-containing caulk must be removed upon discovery"* [19].

THE CONUNDRUM

The EPA's interpretation of TSCA is that if PCB in caulking (or presumably other building materials) is found at levels exceeding 50 ppm, it must be removed. This is clear from the 2005 letter to Kaplowitz and the EPA Fact Sheet entitled,

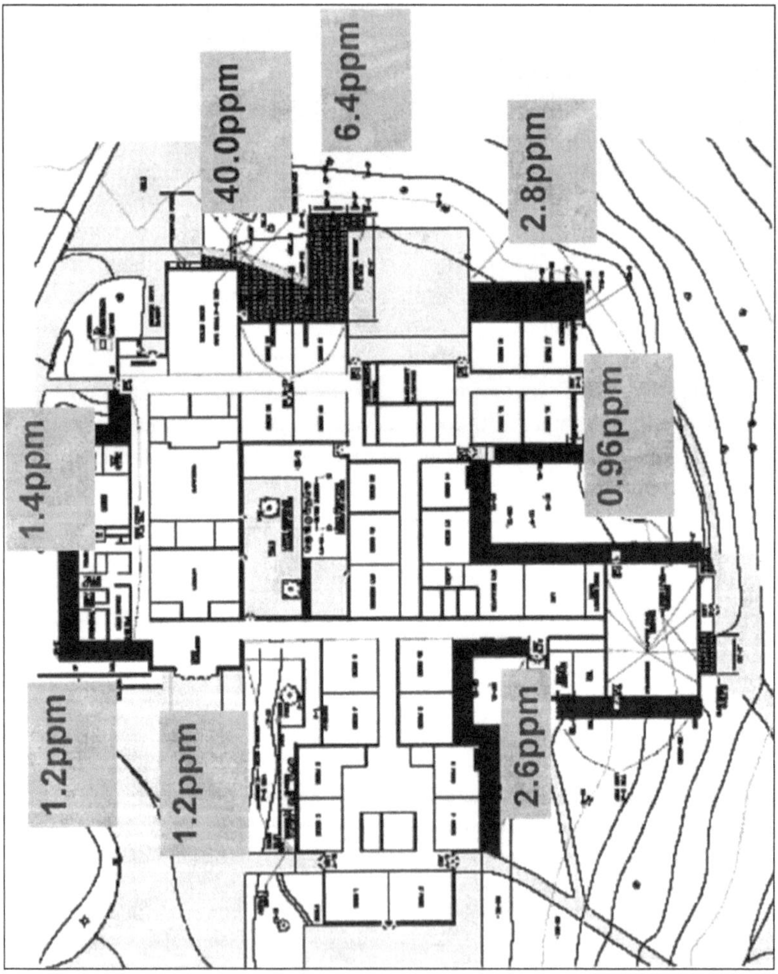

Figure 1. PCB soil contamination, French Hill School, Yorktown Heights, New York.

"Current Best Practices for PCBs in Caulk (updated June 2009)" [20], which states that "caulk containing PCBs at levels > 50 ppm is not authorized for use under the PCB regulations and must be removed." In the case of the university administration building described earlier, the cost of abatement of a 10-story building was approximately $2 million. And while the regulations are clear about the need for removal of PCB-contaminated material upon discovery, there is no requirement that testing be done to find such materials. So what would motivate a building owner to test for PCB contamination in the first place?

So upon this conundrum, things sat for months. On the scientific side, research continued, with another study that showed that PCB soil contamination was possible even when caulking material was intact and undisturbed, and that PCB could be readily mobilized from old caulk by natural weathering [21]. Dr. Lefkowitz continued to push for action to remove the PCB caulk from his son's school and to broaden the investigation to similar buildings.

Dr. Lefkowitz also reached out to a reporter at the *New York Daily News*, Bill Egbert, following which the paper decided to sample caulk at a limited number of schools in New York City. The *Daily News* obtained samples from nine schools and sent them to a state-certified laboratory. Six of the nine samples contained more than the EPA's threshold proportion of 50 ppm PCBs—indeed, at two schools, the levels were literally thousands of times higher: 225,000 at PS 199 in Manhattan and 111,000 ppm at PS 178 in the Bronx. The paper ran a series of stories discussing the discovery, the community response, and a subsequent City Council hearing devoted to the issue. The New York City Department of Education responded to the concern expressed by parents and political leaders by conducting a series of widely criticized tests in the schools in the *Daily News* study and by minimizing the risk of exposure [22].

The *Daily News* series prompted two legal developments. The first one was legislative: New York State Assemblywoman Linda Rosenthal, whose district includes PS 199, the school where the caulk had tested highest for PCBs, sponsored a bill that would mandate testing of the caulk at all New York City schools built during the period when PCBs were in use as plasticizers. The bill garnered the support of a number of co-sponsors but was stalled during the chaos that characterized the New York State Legislature in summer 2009. It will be reintroduced during the next session.

In addition, New York Lawyers for the Public Interest (NYLPI), a civil rights non-profit with an environmental justice section, started a campaign around the issue with two components, community organizing and a litigation. NYLPI filed a formal notice of intent to sue NYC on behalf of Bronx mother Naomi Gonzalez in March 2009; after the notice was filed, the City started meeting with the EPA to discuss the problem of PCB-contaminated caulk. In January 2010, several months after the lawsuit itself was filed in federal court, the City reached agreements with both the EPA and the plaintiff. It will conduct a pilot study to assess the problem's scope and potential remedies, ultimately generating a citywide plan. On a parallel track, in September 2009 EPA headquarters announced new national guidances on PCBs in schools and two major research initiatives.

LABOR'S ROLE

The investigation in the U.S. would never have progressed without the support of labor organizations. The retired bricklayer who identified potentially contaminated buildings in Boston was trained in industrial hygiene principles as part of a program at the CPWR (formerly the Center to Protect Workers' Rights, now the Center for Construction Research and Training). The initial survey that discovered elevated PCB caulking levels in eight of 24 buildings was supported by the International Union of Bricklayers and Allied Craft Workers, Local 3, Eastern Massachusetts. Construction trade workers participated in the first study done in the United States that demonstrated substantial differences in PCB serum levels between construction workers and general population samples. These findings strongly suggest that occupational contact with caulking material can be a major source of PCB exposure for construction workers [23].

More recently, the Massachusetts Teachers Association (MTA) has expressed interest in evaluating the extent to which schools may contain PCB building materials and the possible effect these PCBs may have on their members. The MTA and investigators from Harvard School of Public Health are addressing these questions.

THE WAY FORWARD

Until it posted a Web site on PCB in building caulk in 2008 [24], the U.S. EPA appeared to be in a state of vincible ignorance on the subject. Although PCBs are the only chemicals specifically mentioned in the "Toxic Substances Control Act," and in 1996 the EPA clearly was aware that building caulk could contaminate the interior of buildings [9], the agency seemed willfully ignorant of the problem. In fact, a telephone survey of the 10 EPA regions conducted in 2007 showed a great deal of variability between regions. Regions 1 (Boston), 2 (New York), and 8 (Denver) reported activity on PCB in buildings and other structures, while some others seemed to have little awareness that PCB in building materials was an issue [25]. With the arrival of new leaders in 2009, the EPA has acted to develop guidelines on caulking as a source of PCBs in schools. This guidance represents a promising start, while the effect it will have in practice is yet to be seen. In its September 25, 2009 press release, the EPA stated that ". . . unfortunately high levels of PCBs are present in many buildings and facilities constructed prior to the PCB ban, including most recently some schools. We're concerned about the potential risks associated with exposure to these PCBs . . ." [26]; however, the underlying conundrum in the TSCA regulation remains: There is no requirement that a building owner test for PCB in caulking. But if the owner or another concerned party such as a labor organization or a parent tests for PCB and finds it, TSCA requires that it be removed. In the case of Berkshire (Massachusetts) Community College that did the right thing and tested for PCB in caulk before starting a renovation project, the cost of the project more than doubled from $2.2M to an estimated $5M [27].

Can cash-strapped school districts reasonably be expected to take on the economic burden of addressing PCBs in their buildings? In some cases, renovations that are already planned could easily double in cost, but, in many school districts, needed renovations such as window replacements have been deferred for years. Our data suggests that if testing is done, approximately one-third of the schools constructed from about 1950 to the late 1970s will be found to contain PCBs. To comply with TSCA, these PCBs must be removed or the schools could risk severe penalties, should the EPA pursue enforcement. The only reasonable course to protect teachers, staff, and students from what the EPA acknowledges is a source of concern is to provide federal financial support for PCB testing and removal. House Bill 2187, the "21st Century Green High-Performing Public School Facilities Act" providing such support, was passed on May 18, 2009 by the U.S. House of Representatives and sent to the U.S. Senate Committee on Health, Education, Labor and Pensions. This legislation provides "grants . . . for the purpose of modernizing, renovating, or repairing public school facilities, based on their need for such improvements, to be safe, healthy, high-performing, and up-to-date technologically" [28]. Under allowable uses of funds, this legislation specifies that the grants shall be used for modernization, renovation, or repair of public school facilities, including, where applicable, early learning facilities, including "abatement, removal, or interim controls of asbestos, polychlorinated biphenyls, mold, mildew, or lead-based hazards, including lead-based paint hazards."

CONCLUSIONS

This story has no conclusion; however, there are several undisputable facts:

- Masonry buildings constructed or renovated between about 1950 and the late 1970s may contain PCBs in materials such as caulking and paint, sometimes in very high concentrations.
- PCBs are being released from these materials, contaminating the building interiors and the soil around these buildings.
- Occupants of these buildings may have significantly elevated serum PCB levels, particularly for the more volatile PCB congeners.
- The potential risk from this source of PCB exposure has not been determined; however, there is growing evidence that some of the more volatile PCB congeners released from caulk can be potent neurotoxins [29].
- The EPA has signaled that they intend to strengthen chemical management laws by making changes in TSCA. Specifically, they have identified initiating rulemaking under section 6 of TSCA to re-evaluate the TSCA PCB use and

distribution in commerce regulations as a topic for action [30]. This offers the hope that they will develop a rational public policy to minimize PCB exposure from what appears to be a very significant source.

ACKNOWLEDGMENTS

The contributions of Miranda K. S. Massie, Senior Staff Attorney, New York Lawyers for the Public Interest, are gratefully acknowledged.

REFERENCES

1. U.S. Environmental Protection Agency, "PCBs in Fluorescent Light Fixtures," http://yosemite.epa.gov/R10/EXTAFF.NSF/84c2eal918cf8b90882566e200738f51/8078cb9ed319d3ed882568870002645e/$FILE/pcbfacts.pdf (accessed September 30, 2009).
2. California Department of Toxic Substances Control, "Fact Sheet—PCBs in Schools," http://www.dtsc.ca.gov/Schools/upload/SM_FS_PCB_Schools.pdf (accessed September 30, 2009).
3. Chr. Benthe et al., "Polychlorinated Biphenyls. Indoor Air Contamination Due to Thiokol-Rubber Sealants in an Office Building," *Chemosphere* (1992): 1481-1486.
4. E. Balfanz, J. Fuchs, and H. Kieper, "Sampling and Analysis of Polychlorinated Biphenyls (PCB) in Indoor Air due to Permanently Elastic Sealants," *Chemosphere* 26, (1993) 5: 871-880.
5. U. Burkhardt et al., "Indoor Air Pollution by Polychlorinated Biphenyl Compounds in Permanently Elastic Sealants," *Offentl Gesundheitweis* 52, (1990) 10: 567-574.
6. R. Corner et al., "PCB in Indoor Air and Dust in Buildings in Stockholm," in *Indoor Air 2002*, proceedings from the 9th International Conference on Indoor Air Quality and Climate, Monterey, California, June 30–July 5 (2002) 4: 141-146.
7. H. Fromme et al., "Polychlorinated Biphenyls (PCB) in Caulking Compounds of Buildings-Assessment of Current Status in Berlin and New Indoor Air Sources," *Gesundheitswesen* 58, (1996) 12: 666-672.
8. V. Pyy and O. Lyly, *PCB in Jointing Materials in Prefabricated Houses and in the Soil of Yards* (Helsinki, Finland: City of Helsinki Environment Centre, 1998).
9. "Use Authorization for, and Distribution in Commerce of, Non- liquid Polychlorinated Biphenyls; Notice of Availability; Partial Reopening of Comment Period," *Federal Register* 64, 237 (December 10, 1999).
10. S. Leung, "Source of Toxin Revealed at Bourne School," *Boston Globe*, March 21, 1996.
11. F. Neisel et al., "Human Biomonitoring of Polychlorinated Biphenyls in 130 Exposed Elementary School Children," *Gesundheitswesen* 61, (1999) 3: 137-149
12. T. Gabrio et al., "PCB-Blood Levels in Teachers, Working in PCB-Contaminated Schools," *Chemosphere* 40, (2000) 9-11: 1055-1062.
13. M. Schwenk et al., "Human Biomonitoring of Polychlorinated Biphenyls and Polychlorinated Dibenzodioxins and Dibenzofuranes in Teachers Working in a PCB-Contaminated School," *Chemosphere* 47, (2002) 2: 229-233.
14. B. Liebel et al., "Evidence for Increased Internal Exposure to Lower Chlorinated Polychlorinated Biphenyls (PCB) in Pupils Attending a Contaminated School," *International Journal of Hygiene and Environmental Health*, 237 (2004): 315-324.

15. K. Coghlan et al., "Characterization of Polychlorinated Biphenyls in Building Materials and Exposures in the Indoor Environment," in *Indoor Air 2002*, proceedings from the 9th International Conference on Indoor Air Quality and Climate, Monterey, California, June 30–July 5 (2002) 4, 147-152.
16. M. Chang, K. Coghlan, and J. McCarthy, "Remediating PCB-Containing Building Products: Strategies and Regulatory Considerations," in *Indoor Air 2002*, proceedings from the 9th International Conference on Indoor Air Quality and Climate, Monterey, California, June 30–July 5 (2002) 4: 171-176.
17. E. Priha, "Health and Environmental Aspects of PCB Contamination Due to Old Polysulfide Sealants," from podium session 104, presentation no. 25, American Industrial Hygiene Conference and Exposition, Dallas, Texas (May 2003).
18. Author, 2004.
19. U.S. Environmental Protection Agency, Letter to Michael Kaplowitz, November 3, 2005, http://www.pcbinschools.org/EPA%20LETTER.pdf accessed September 30, 2009.
20. U.S. Environmental Protection Agency, "Current Best Practices for PCBs in Caulk Fact Sheet: Removal and Clean-Up of PCBs in Caulk and PCB-Contaminated Soil and Building Material," http://www.epa.gov/pcbsincaulk/caulkremoval.htm (accessed September 30, 2009).
21. Author, 2007.
22. Testimony of Kathleen Grimm, Deputy Chancellor, Finance and Administration, New York City Department of Education, New York City Council Committees on Education, Environmental Protection, and Oversight and Investigations Special Hearing on PCBs in Schools, April 29, 2008.
23. Author, 2007.
24. U.S. Environmental Protection Agency, "PCBs in Caulk in Older Buildings," http://www.epa.gov/waste/hazard/tsd/pcbs/pubs/caulk/index.htm (accessed September 30, 2009).
25. M. Parks, research report submitted in partial fulfillment of M.S. degree requirements, Harvard School of Public Health, May, 2007.
26. U.S. Environmental Protection Agency, "EPA Announces Guidance to Communities on PCBs in Caulk of Buildings Constructed or Renovated Between 1950 and 1978: EPA to gather latest science on PCBs in caulk," http://yosemite.epa.gov/opa/admpress.nsf/d0cf6618525a9efb85257359003fb69d/28c8384eea0e67ed8525763c005 9342f!OpenDocument (accessed September 30, 2009).
27. J. Smith, "Berkshire Community College Cleanup to cost $5M," *Berkshire Eagle*, Sept. 5, 2009.
28. *21st Century Green High-Performing Public School Facilities Act*, HR 2187, http://thomas.loc.gov/cgi-bin/bdquery/z?d111:HR02187 (accessed September 30, 2009).
29. T. Simon, J. Britt, and R. James, "Development of a Neurotoxic Equivalence Scheme of Relative Potency for Assessing the Risk of PCB Mixtures," *Regul Toxicol Pharmacol* 48 (2007) 2: 148-170.
30. U.S. Environmental Protection Agency, "Enhancing EPA's Chemical Management Program," http://www.epa.gov/oppt/existingchemicals/pubs/enhanchems.html (accessed September 30, 2009).

Update on PCBs in School

Robert F. Herrick

The public health challenge posed by polychlorinated biphenyls (PCBs) in schools (and other buildings) remains largely unaddressed in 2013. The overall level of awareness has increased as the National Institute for Occupational Safety and Health (NIOSH), the U.S. Environmental Protection Agency (EPA), state and local governments, professional and trade associations, unions, consultants, and law firms have spread the word. NIOSH addressed the findings that teachers in PCB-containing schools, and construction trade workers renovating these buildings, can have elevated serum PCB levels as a result of these occupational exposures [1]. In some regions (specifically New England and New York), building renovations that involve disturbing or removing caulk, sealants, or paint now include testing for PCBs (as well as lead and asbestos) before work is conducted. When PCBs are found, they are removed following abatement procedures that are similar to those used for lead or asbestos. The conundrum mentioned earlier (testing is not required, but if testing finds PCBs at concentrations exceeding 50 ppm, it is a Toxic Substances Control Act (TSCA) violation) has not been resolved. Some state departments of education have adopted protocols that recommend testing before building renovations that involve disturbing PCB caulk, paint, and other materials [2], and the National Aeronautics and Space Administration [3] has policies requiring testing for PCBs prior to renovations or demolitions. EPA Regional Offices have approved a variety of approaches to remove, encapsulate, and contain PCB sources in buildings [4].

Probably the most noteworthy recent development is the finding that PCB-containing fluorescent light fixtures are still common in schools, and they are contributing to indoor PCB contamination. When the City of New York reached an agreement with EPA Region 2 on PCB caulking in New York City schools, the city undertook a pilot study to evaluate the presence of PCB caulk, and to investigate alternative approaches to remediation (Consent Agreement and Final Order [CAFO], Docket Number TSCA-02-2010-9201) [5]. The pilot study included air sampling, and a substantial number of schools were found to have PCB air levels that exceeded EPA guidelines [6], in some cases by large factors (levels up to 1,000 ng PCB/m^3 reported; EPA guidelines range from 70 to 600 ng/m^3, depending upon the age of children in the school). Upon further investigation, the presence of PCB caulk was confirmed, but fluorescent lights in these schools were also found with magnetic light ballasts that contained

PCBs [5]. Many of these light ballasts had failed, releasing PCBs into the school buildings. The fact that so many ballasts had failed cannot be surprising, as these fluorescent lights were typically installed in the period from 1950 until the mid- to late1970s, and these ballasts have an estimated lifetime of 10 to 15 years [7]. It is surprising, however, that so many of these antiquated lights are still in service. The final results of the pilot study are still being analyzed, but it seems clear that elevated PCB levels in building air can be attributed to multiple sources (including caulk, paint, leaking light ballasts, and possibly others such as carpet adhesives, fireproofing, and ceiling tiles). Remediation efforts to reduce PCB exposures to occupants of these buildings will therefore require a comprehensive approach to identify these multiple sources.

Although most of the U.S. activity on PCB-containing buildings has been conducted in New England and New York, there is no reason to conclude that PCBs are confined to buildings in this region. An investigation conducted in the San Francisco Bay area, for example, collected 25 caulk samples from the exterior of 10 buildings. PCBs were detected in 88 percent of the caulk samples, at concentrations ranging from 1 to 220,000 ppm; 40 percent exceeded the EPA threshold of 50 ppm. These investigators concluded that PCBs are prevalent in currently standing Bay Area buildings constructed during the period of PCB usage [8].

Finally, PCB testing remains controversial. In New York City, for example, elected officials from across the city, and a number of groups including New York Communities for Change, New York Lawyers for the Public Interest, representatives from the United Federation of Teachers (UFT), 32BJ, Laborers International Union of North America (LIUNA) Local 78, other labor organizations, and parents, demanded that the New York City Department of Education (DOE) rid all NYC schools of PCBs. When EPA conducted spot inspections at nine NYC public schools in the winter of 2010-2011, PCB-leaking light fixtures were found at 100 percent of the school buildings and in 93 percent of the locations inspected. DOE responded by instituting a visual inspection program, which has resulted in more than 400 schools being fast-tracked for complete PCB light replacement within one year. DOE, however, has told parents at the remaining 783 schools with PCB lights that they must wait up to nine years before DOE will replace the PCB lights in their children' school. In response, a coalition including legislators, advocacy groups, and citizens has requested that EPA Region 2 re-institute its spot inspection program.

In May 2013, the DOE and the NYC School Construction Authority agreed to a settlement requiring that all PCB light fixtures be removed by December 31, 2016 [9].

In other cases, the right of workers and their representatives to request testing and inspections for PCBs in buildings, or to conduct testing on their own, has been challenged by building owners. As a result, the extent to which people live, work, or attend school in PCB-contaminated buildings is unknown. Until there is a well-designed national survey of buildings constructed or renovated from

1950 to 1980, which we called for in 2004 [10], there will not be a rational policy to reduce the potentially significant health risks resulting from these sources of PCB exposure.

NOTES

1. http://www.cdc.gov/niosh/docs/2012-170/ (accessed August 15, 2012).
2. http://www.p12.nysed.gov/facplan/HealthSafety/PCBinCaulkProtocol-070615.html
3. http://environmental.ksc.nasa.gov/permitting/wastePcb.htm, http://www.nasa.gov/pdf/510315main_Close%20Demolish%20Facilities%20Structures,%20Direct%20Project%2097963.4%20Rev%204.pdf,
4. D. L. MacIntosh et al., "Mitigation of Building-Related Polychlorinated Biphenyls in Indoor Air of a School," *Environmental Health* 11 (2012): 24.
5. http://www.nycsca.org/Community/Programs/EPA-NYC-PCB/Pages/default.aspx
6. http://www.epa.gov/pcbsincaulk/maxconcentrations.pdf
7. http://www.epa.gov/epawaste/hazard/tsd/pcbs/pubs/ballasts.htm
8. S. Klosterhaus, D. Yee, J. Kass, A. Wong, and L. McKee, *PCBs in Caulk Project: Estimated Stock in Currently Standing Buildings in a San Francisco Bay Study Area and Releases to Stormwater during Renovation and Demolition* (SFEI Contribution 651), 2011, San Francisco Estuary Institute, Oakland, CA.
9. http://www.nylpi.org/
10. R. F. Herrick et al., "An Unrecognized Source of PCB Contamination in Schools and Other Buildings," *Environmental Health Perspectives* 112(10) (2004): 1051-1053.

CHAPTER 5

Healthy School Siting and Planning Policies: Linking Public Health, Education, and the Environment

Alison K. Cohen

Policy decisions regarding the quality of the physical school environment—both school siting and school facility planning policies—are often considered through the lens of environmental planning, public health, or education policy, but rarely through all three. Environmental planners consider environmental justice issues on a local level and/or consider the regional impact of a school. Public health professionals focus on toxic exposures and populations particularly vulnerable to negative health outcomes. Educators and education policymakers emphasize investing in human capital of both students and staff. By understanding these respective angles and combining these efforts around the common goals of achieving adequacy and excellence, we can work toward a regulatory system for school facilities that recognizes children as a uniquely vulnerable population and seeks to create healthier school environments in which children can learn and adults can work.

WHY SHOULD WE CARE ABOUT THE PHYSICAL SCHOOL ENVIRONMENT?

Questions about the quality of the physical school environment have historically been overlooked, and research is just beginning to emerge regarding the connections and potential for collaboration among urban planning, health, and academic outcomes [1]. Research is especially important because 20 percent of Americans (students and staff combined) go to school every day [2, 3], and schools are a critical component of urban infrastructure [4]. Students spend over 1,300 hours in school facilities annually (second only to the amount of time spent at home), but approximately 50 percent of all public schools—and disproportionately urban schools and schools serving low-income students or students of color—have at least one "unsatisfactory environmental condition" [5]. According to data from 1998, the average age of a school building was 42 years, with three-quarters of schools built before 1970, when lead paint was commonly used [2]. The quality of school facilities is a critical, but understudied, education issue.

This article analyzes three disciplines that have a stake in the physical school environment—environmental planning, public health, and education policy—and explores how and why each discipline engages in school facility policy, as an updated version of an article published in 2010 [6]. Environmental planners have considered how the physical school environment fits into larger regional planning endeavors, as well as some of the environment impacts and implications associated with the quality of the land and facility. Public health scholars have demonstrated that environmentally healthy schools lead to healthier students who perform better in school and that school facilities have a larger impact on student performance than commonly accepted factors such as student attitudes toward learning [7]. Education policymakers consider how investments in school infrastructure will increase the human capital of the students and staff learning and working there. A brief content analysis of support letters sent to the House Committee on Education and Labor regarding a school facility bill introduces the perspectives of various stakeholders. An application of these lenses to illustrative examples of major lawsuits and relevant research endeavors follows. Given the limited research on school siting and school building, these examples are dispersed across the country and provide diverse entry points to the issue.

WHO CARES ABOUT THE PHYSICAL SCHOOL ENVIRONMENT?

The multitude and variety of supporters of the 21st Century High-Performing Public Schools Facilities Act, which was passed by the House in May 2009 with the goal of modernizing school buildings to make them more efficient, illustrate the types of stakeholders involved in and/or affected by school planning decisions. Groups publicly supporting the Act included: school professional associations (including the American Federation of Teachers and the National Education Association), labor unions/professional associations (including the Building and Construction Trades Department of the AFL-CIO and the International Union of Painters and Allied Trades), environmentalists (including Environment America and the U.S. Green Building Council), and groups devoted to school facility improvement (including Rebuilding America's Schools and Californians for School Facilities) [8].

The official letters of support submitted to Representative George Miller, chair of the House Committee on Education and Labor, in reference to the 21st Century

High-Performing Public School Facilities Act highlight the different ways in which stakeholders are affected by school facility planning decisions. (All these letters are available on the following website (accessed 16 Sept. 2008): http://edlabor.house.gov/issues/schoolfacilitiesact.shtml). In a qualitative analysis of the content of each of the 18 letters, four different rationales for support for the bill emerged: the environment, health, education, and the economy. Not surprisingly, as this bill originated in the Education and Labor Committee, all 18 letters mentioned the benefits of the legislation for education, including raising student achievement. Most commonly, letters referred to new facilities helping to improve student achievement. Similarly, and perhaps due to the nature of the committee's dual focus on education and labor, six letters were from associations of builders or tradesmen, and 15 of the 18 letters discussed the benefits of the bill on economic development. In particular, these arguments focused on the creation of new jobs through investment in infrastructure, with only four of the letters mentioning preparing students for future economic success. The environment and health were much less frequently mentioned. Seven letters mentioned benefits for the environment, namely energy efficiency and the use of renewable resources, and only three mentioned potential health benefits—that this legislation would help all school facilities meet basic health and safety codes. This snapshot of the stakeholder positions on a single school facility bill underscores the emphasis on economic and education outcomes, in line with the mandate of the committee, and a relative de-emphasis on the environment and health. The research body, on the other hand, emphasizes environment and health as key components of school planning policies. Researchers and policymakers should collaborate to consider how to overlap to support research-informed policy.

The diversity of stakeholders in healthy school facility policy decisions is complicated by the lack of communication and lack of analytical overlap in methods: city planners rarely talk to education professionals, and neither is likely to learn about school siting or facility planning in their professional training [9]. The review of environmental plans tends to be confined to particular technical levels of analysis and compartmentalizes the impact of certain discipline-specific regulatory decisions [10]. This makes it more difficult to understand and address the variety of stakeholders and policy realms that a particular siting decision may affect.

WHY DO ENVIRONMENTAL PLANNERS CARE ABOUT THE PHYSICAL SCHOOL ENVIRONMENT?

In a 1955 commentary about community planning and education, Francis Violich remarked, "without the land itself, and with any [physical] conditions lacking, the ability of the educational plant to serve human needs is impaired" [11]. Over the past 50-plus years, public education has changed in many ways, but the reliance on adequate land and physical conditions remains. There are two major sources of environmental problems in schools: the quality of the land on which the school is built, and the quality of the school facility itself. Environmental planners use two lenses to tackle these two issues: focusing on the local environment of the particular facility and focusing on the regional environment of the larger area in which the facility is located. The facility focus considers the quality of the school environment and how the facility is managed. From a school staff perspective, this is where teachers and especially custodial staff may be involved. The facility focus considers questions of environmental injustices affecting a particular school's student and staff population. The regional focus considers how the quality of the school may affect or influence other buildings and developments in the neighborhood, city, or region, often within the context of building social capital.

The Local Environment: Environmental Justice

Around the country, including in Providence, Rhode Island, people have raised concerns about the environmental quality of a particular school facility and how it affects the people at that school; and it is primarily environmental planners and managers who have worked to address these questions. Often, these schools are located in low-income communities or communities of color, raising questions of environmental justice. On a basic level, environmental justice is the right of all people (regardless of race, class, or background) to live, work, play, and learn in a safe and healthy environment [12, 13]. The environmental justice movement integrates concerns about the environment, health, and civil rights to consider the disproportionate environmental pollution and health burden that disenfranchised communities—primarily low-income communities and communities of color—bear [14]. The Environmental Protection Agency defines environmental justice specifically as the "fair treatment and meaningful involvement" of all people in the "development, implementation, and enforcement" of environmental policies and regulations [15]. However, school facilities may perpetuate environmental injustice in two ways.

First, schools may be sited on contaminated land, or on a brownfield. Brownfields are properties that are contaminated or believed to be contaminated and that are being underused or not used at all [16]. In many Northeastern cities (including Providence, Rhode Island), land is scarce, and most land parcels available for building are brownfields [17]. Brownfields tend to be located in poorer communities and low-income communities of color [16, 18]. At the same time, however, poorer districts are more likely to be overcrowded and in need of new schools [19]. Building a school on a brownfield may be the only way in which a school can be proximal to the students it serves [20]. Schools may also be sited near environmental polluters. Grade schools located closer to environmental hazards in a Florida school district were disproportionately black and Hispanic and more highly segregated, while schools located further away were disproportionately white [21]. Similarly, schools that serve primarily students of color are more likely to have higher rates of exposure to hazardous air pollutants and have a higher risk of associated health problems [22]. The frequency of building schools on brownfields is an environmental justice issue that has only recently gained traction, despite how critical it is to ensuring healthy school environments.

Second, schools may themselves be in sub-par condition. Fifty percent of all public schools—and disproportionately urban schools and schools serving low-income students or students of color—have at least one "unsatisfactory environmental condition," including ventilation and heating problems [5]. The General Accounting Office (now General Accountability Office) determined in 1995 that one-third of all public school facilities were in a "serious state of disrepair"; a 2000 National Education Association report estimates this will cost $322 billion to redress [9]. Facilities in disrepair are concentrated in urban areas that tend to serve students of low socioeconomic status [1].

The Regional Perspective: Neighborhood Quality and Community Development

Not all environmental planners operate on the level of an individual school. Some, who emphasize neighborhood quality and community development, consider how school facilities may affect the quality of the greater community's built environment, and how the quality of the school—whether it be poorly maintained or an exercise in innovation and urban renewal—makes the neighborhood more or less desirable.

The quality of the school affects perceptions about the quality of the neighborhood. A well-maintained school not only makes it a healthier place for students to learn, but it affects perceptions about the surrounding neighborhood; a poorly maintained school or a school located close to a polluter can be less desirable, making the neighborhood a less desirable place to live [21]. Vincent argues that public schools offer both a "physical and social" infrastructure, so that, in addition to the actual property investment, schools can help build a community's social environment [9]. The concept of a social infrastructure means that healthy schools have the potential to contribute to healthy communities. In poorer districts with the double problem of brownfields and school overcrowding, building new schools on remediated brownfields can help revitalize a neighborhood by reducing perceived blight [23]. Alternatively, if the brownfields are left unremediated before school construction begins, or if the construction site is left fallow for an extended period of time, perceived blight can persist in the neighborhood.

School quality is a motivating force in driving people out of cities and into suburbs, leading to residential and school re-segregation [24, 25]. As planners try to counteract sprawl with "smart growth" initiatives, they must also consider urban education policies. For example, Maryland's Smart Growth planners prioritize school rehabilitation to begin to address underlying education issues, including racial desegregation in schools and working toward smaller, community-centered schools [24]. Leadership in Energy and Environmental Design (LEED)-certified schools can be beacons of innovation in a community and encourage both people and innovation to concentrate in the community. However, LEED certification and green design are only beginning to catch on across the country. Only 13 percent of districts currently have policies to include green design principles in school construction projects [2]. Furthermore, LEED standards focus more on reducing resource consumption than on reducing hazardous exposures, with only one category (indoor environmental quality) explicitly addressing such potential exposures. While brownfields remediation and upgrading to achieving LEED certification do not have to be mutually exclusive solutions for creating healthier school environments, the Providence case study described below reveals that typically only one of these methods is offered as a solution, depending on where the school is located and what population the school serves.

Environmental Adequacy and Environmental Excellence

Environmental Adequacy: Brownfields

Two examples of brownfields remediation for schools—the Triad Approach used in New Jersey and the Child Proofing Our Communities approach recommended by the Center for Health and Environmental Justice—focus on ensuring safety. The Triad Approach is one approach used to identify whether a site is suitable for construction. It was used in New Jersey to characterize the environmental quality of a brownfields site that was identified as the potential location of an elementary school that needed to be built to help reduce overcrowding [19]. Endorsed by the U.S. Environmental Protection Agency (EPA) and the New Jersey Department of Environmental Protection, the Triad Approach describes the conditions of the site to help reduce the amount of time it takes to construct a new school, something that has been an explicit goal of the state of New Jersey [19, 26]. The Triad Approach to brownfields remediation offers a policy solution to a common problem of the brownfields remediation process—that city officials get permits without doing background research about the environmental quality of the site [23]. There are three components of the Triad: strategic planning, dynamic work strategies that allow the project to be completed more rapidly and less expensively, and real-time measurement technologies that make rapid data collection possible [27]. By using field analysis methods, scientists collecting environmental samples to determine contamination levels can analyze their samples on-site, which makes it easier to collect more samples in a more targeted and thorough manner [26].

The Triad Approach also expedites the entire data collection process: At one New Jersey school site, only two months elapsed between the preliminary site visit and the analysis of the data collected; the process typically takes twice as long [19, 26]. The Triad Approach's emphasis on expedited review and the role of highly specialized professionals in collecting the data circumvent extensive community engagement in the planning process, since meaningful community engagement requires additional time and resources and an emphasis on specialization simultaneously deemphasizes the importance of local knowledge. Triad Approach data may be strong, but it is not disseminated at the community level. Just 17 states require school planners to open up their plans for public comment [20]. This is a potential barrier to environmental equity because the regulatory decision-making process often overlooks questions of disproportionate pollution burden and environmental justice, so when community members' opinions about the site go unheard, so, too, do these concerns. Not only is involvement in the regulatory process a key tenet of the environmental justice movement, but it is also something that residents in minority neighborhoods are interested in: three-quarters of study respondents in a minority neighborhood with many brownfields expressed a desire to participate in the redevelopment process [1].

The Child Proofing Our Communities Campaign (CPOC), an initiative by the Center for Health, Environment, and Justice, developed model federal school siting legislation. Its essential components are: ensuring public participation in the decision-making process by having a citizen group that democratically decides upon the progression of the project, categorically denying the use of some sites due to particularly harmful environmental pollution present, and conducting a thorough environmental hazard and health assessment. Then, if a contaminated site must be used, CPOC advocates for developing and implementing a remediation plan that includes certain key steps, such as minimizing exposure to contaminated soil and developing a system to vent volatile organic chemicals [20].

Environmental Excellence: High-Performance Schools

At the first Rhode Island Sustainable Schools Summit in September 2008, multiple panelists, who came both from the sustainability movement and from school planning and facilities management, focused on building and renovating schools to the highest environmental standards as the way to achieve healthy and sustainable schools. High-performance schools have societal benefits in addition to benefits for the individuals attending: they can help the environment and reduce costs by being more energy-efficient, freeing up other funds for important policy priorities [3]. The highest environmental standards most often used are the U.S. Green Building Council's LEED (Leadership in Energy and Environmental Design) rating system, which was originally designed as a tool to change the market for commercial buildings but has quickly been taken up in the public sector and government as well [28]. Key components of the general LEED certification process include: the choice of site (with points offered for redeveloping and reusing existing sites); water-use reduction and efficiency; renewable and efficient energy use; waste reduction, reuse, and recycling; improving the quality of the indoor environment (air, temperature, physical space, etc.); and innovative design features [28].

As of 2006, the U.S. Green Building Council (USGBC) reported that seven federal agencies, 11 states, and 43 cities had legislation or incentives that encouraged the development of LEED-certified buildings [29, 30]. The USGBC launched a nationwide initiative to work with state lawmakers to promote green schools to increase the number of green schools across the country (USGBC has currently registered over 1,000) [31]. State laws vary widely, ranging from little or no regulation to examples such as Washington state's High Performance Public Building Act of 2005. The Act requires all Washington state public school facility projects receiving state funding to achieve at least the LEED silver standard or follow the Washington Sustainable Schools Design Protocol [32]. The Washington Sustainable Schools Protocol was developed by a 34-member committee that included nine representatives from public school districts across the state, nine members of architecture and/or engineering firms, seven government representatives (four from the office of the superintendent for public instruction, three from others), two representatives of public utilities, two interior designers, four members from energy efficiency groups, and one sustainable design consultant [33], signaling the diversity of perspectives within the realm of environmental planning and design. Washington's policy and similar policies in other states engage many types of public planners, but their greatest limitation is that they apply only for the creation of new facilities and do little, if anything, to address issues with existing buildings.

A Tale of Two Schools in Providence, Rhode Island

The two policy solutions of brownfields remediation and LEED certification/energy efficiency described above offer different approaches for improving the school environment. In Providence, both approaches have been used, in two neighborhoods serving two different populations. Brownfields remediation focuses on achieving environmental adequacy, whereas LEED certification and efficiency focus on environmental excellence. Given this distinction, brownfields remediation tends to be a policy most commonly considered in urban areas and low-income communities, where brownfields are concentrated. Here, the environmental planning focus is on ensuring that the school environment causes no harm. On the other hand, LEED certification is optional and requires more funding, so is most commonly considered in wealthier districts. Here, the environmental planning focus is on making the school an even healthier place to be.

In the case of brownfields, Anthony Carnevale Elementary School and Springfield Middle School ("the Springfield Street schools") were built upon Providence's former city dump in the Hartford Park neighborhood in 1999.

Sixty-six percent of Hartford Park's residents are people of color, whereas in Providence as a whole, 55 percent of residents are people of color. The neighborhood is almost 50 percent Hispanic, 20 percent more than Providence as a whole. Forty percent of families are below the poverty level, as compared to 24 percent of Providence residents overall [34, 35]. Over 80 percent of the students attending the two schools were students of color and from low-income families [34]. In 1999, Rhode Island Legal Services filed a lawsuit on behalf of local residents against the R.I. Department of Environmental Management (DEM) alleging that the DEM had violated hazardous waste cleanup laws by approving the school siting and minimal cleanup plan [36]. The civil suit alleged that the plan was environmentally racist and inequitable because a low-income community of color would be disproportionately burdened [37]. While the Rhode Island Superior Court found that the DEM protected students from toxic exposures from the ground pollution, the court ruled that the DEM did not achieve state requirements for environmental equity or community involvement in its rushed approval of Providence's plan [36]. Achieving an adequately clean environment was insufficient, and parents of children in Hartford Park and the greater neighborhood community who were minimally engaged in the planning process argued that they deserved greater access and power in the planning process to determine what their local school should look like. Further analysis by the Brown University Superfund Research Program Community Outreach Core has determined that the Springfield street schools are indicative of larger trends: environmentally burdened schools are most concentrated in Providence's low-income communities and communities of color [37].

Across town, in one of the wealthiest neighborhoods in Providence [38], a different story unfolded. In response to declining enrollments, the Nathan Bishop Middle School on Providence's East Side is currently undergoing a $35 million refurbishment to help make public schooling a more appealing option to families living on the East Side [39]. One article from the *Providence Journal* summed up the situation this way: "After years of white flight to the suburbs, some East Side families are willing to give the public schools another chance, especially now that the city is building a new Nathan Bishop Middle School on the East Side" [40]. After initial plans for its closure, parents of both current and prospective students advocated for the renovation and re-opening of the school. Parents formed the East Side Public Education Committee, a structured advocacy group, and the then-superintendent engaged these parents in the school planning process through a formal advisory committee [39]. This extensive parental and community involvement in the planning process is unusual. One reason why parents may have been more heavily involved here is because of the combined political and economic power they held: parents on the East Side had the socioeconomic flexibility to move to another town with better private schools and/or to send their children to private schools. Additionally, since parents were so involved in the planning process, it follows that they would advocate for a school plan that would improve the quality of their neighborhood. The parent community hopes that environmental improvements such as a rainwater collection system and energy-efficient systems at Nathan Bishop, one of the Providence Preservation Society's Most Endangered Properties in 2007, are part of what will draw families to public schools [41, 42]. Here, the particularly excellent school environment is a "pull" factor for families considering public schools.

These examples explore the two ways in which environmental planners conceptualize the physical school environment: environmental adequacy, as evidenced by the environmental justice approach to brownfields, and neighborhood improvement, as characterized by high-performance schools and schools as beacons for the community. Turning to another group, we explore how public health professionals build upon the framework of environmental justice to consider how people are affected by disproportionate exposure to pollution.

WHY DO PUBLIC HEALTH PROFESSIONALS CARE ABOUT THE PHYSICAL SCHOOL ENVIRONMENT?

The public health perspective is people-oriented: it focuses on how the environment—including how the environment is regulated—affects people's lives. This includes focusing on toxic exposures—environmental exposures known or presumed to cause harm—and a special emphasis on populations especially vulnerable to such exposures who may be disproportionately burdened, including youth. The public health focus on health disparities deepens the environmental justice perspective observed in environmental planning and focuses on the human rights and disparate health implications associated with environmental injustice.

Vulnerable Populations

Vulnerable populations experience greater health effects, given the level of their exposure, than the average person exposed. Depending on who these people are, this can again raise issues of justice and equity. Children are a vulnerable population because they are still developing and are more susceptible to toxicants altering their developmental processes. Children have elevated rates of exposure to environmental hazards because they spend more time on the floor (especially younger children) and put more things in their mouth. Additionally, children breathe in proportionately more air than adults [2]. Once children have been exposed, they can experience different toxicological effects than adults that may be particularly harmful to the brain and other organs due to different absorption and metabolism severity [22]. Young men of color have also been identified as a particularly vulnerable population for health and educational outcomes [43].

Furthermore, health problems with long latency periods will have adequate time to develop in children, whereas they may not have ample time to manifest in adults [2]. In fact, President Clinton issued Executive Order 13045 in 1997 to call for the federal government to consider children's special vulnerability to environmental health risks [44]. Additionally, communities that are already exposed to myriad pollutants in their neighborhood—and such pollution is concentrated in low-income communities of color—are also vulnerable [13].

Toxic Exposures

Environmental exposures are much easier to quantify than health outcomes, so exposures to toxic substances and environmental hazards are often measured as a proxy for quantifying negative health outcomes. Much of the public health literature focuses on where people live, but students may not go to school in the same community in which they live, given the increase in busing and magnet school policies [22]. Since students spend a significant portion of their day in school, it is important to consider the school environment.

School buildings—especially older, more rundown schools—are plagued by a number of environmental health threats, including lead paint, mold, and even asbestos [20]. Lead paint was commonly used in buildings pre-1978, so the risk of lead paint exposure alone can be significant in older school buildings. These dilapidated schools also tend to disproportionately serve low-income communities and communities of color [20].

Indoor air quality of schools is of particular concern: 20 percent of American schools have reported that their indoor air quality is unsatisfactory [45], and one study found schools to have elevated levels of carbon dioxide, humidity, and allergens (such as dust and mold) in the indoor air [2]. Formaldehyde exposure is also a problem, particularly in portable classroom trailers [46]. However, indoor air quality issues have been overlooked by the majority of states: only 10 states, or one-fifth, require districts and schools to prevent and resolve any indoor air quality problems (often using the EPA's Indoor Air Quality Tools for Schools program as a model) [2]. That said, schools are more likely than other buildings to have poor indoor air quality because omnipresent funding problems mean that facilities are often inadequately maintained [47]. Indoor air quality problems may trigger asthma and can lead to fatigue; headaches; and eye, nose, and throat irritations [2]. One study found that almost two-thirds of teachers who were unable to open classroom windows reported health problems, as compared to just over one-third of teachers who were able to open their windows [48]. Pesticides are widely used in schools—especially schools already of poor quality that, for example, offer easy indoor access to pests through cracks in the walls and floors. Students may become acutely ill due to pesticide exposures in their school [49]. These numerous indoor environment issues can cause health problems and distract children from learning.

In addition to having environmental health problems in the schools, schools can also be located near polluters and other sources of toxic exposures. Despite a growing case for concern, only 14 states have policies that restrict or prohibit the siting of schools on or near toxic sites or sources of pollution. Twenty-four states have no policies requiring school planners to assess environmental hazards at sites being considered for new schools, and 20 states have no policies requiring school planners to consider the environment when siting or building a school [20]. Even common sources of pollution pose a health and academic risk to school children [1]. For example, schools located near high-traffic roads have a larger percentage of students of color than schools further from traffic, and living near high-traffic roads is associated with health problems [50]. Others have considered how school assignment may be associated with children's exposure to vehicle emissions during their commute to school [1].

Environmental Health Adequacy and Environmental Health Excellence

Because public health professionals consider the entire population and are concerned about equitable offerings, they have focused almost exclusively on achieving environmental health adequacy for schools, with little attention being paid to environmental health excellence. Unlike the realm of environmental planning, policies and research for the creation and maintenance of particularly healthy schools are rare, if they exist at all, in the field of public health.

Environmental Health Adequacy

In a study with implications for all metropolitan areas, children of color in Los Angeles Unified School District (LAUSD) were at a higher risk for health problems (both noncancer and cancer problems) associated with exposure to air toxics, even when controlling for land use patterns, socioeconomic status, and other potential confounders [22]. For both average lifetime cancer risk and respiratory health risk, Latino, African-American, and Asian students face a higher risk than white students [22]. Students of color bear a disproportionate health burden due to differential environmental exposures, a clear environmental injustice.

Air pollution increases health problems, primarily respiratory problems, which can in turn lead to reduced academic performance [51]. On the school level, exposure to environmental hazards (as measured by proximity to a Toxic Release Inventory site) is associated with decreased academic performance [51]. Most data regarding academic performance is aggregated on the school level. Schools with the highest exposures to respiratory hazards perform significantly lower on school-level measures of academic performance (the relationship is linear and dose-response), and students of color are more likely to attend schools with higher risks of health problems related to air pollution [44]. Problems of toxic exposures affecting particularly vulnerable populations in schools can be further explored in the case study of the Belmont school in Los Angeles.

Environmental Health Excellence

Evidence is emerging around environmental health excellence for schools, including through community gardens [1] and walkable schools [52], but the research base remains sparse and aspirational.

A Tale of Countless Schools

The construction of the Belmont Learning Complex in Los Angeles was proposed to address overcrowding in a primarily Latino neighborhood [53]. However, the school was built on top of a heavily contaminated former oil field. Although the Los Angeles Unified School District knew about the presence of toxic chemicals on the site, it kept quiet about the problem to speed up the construction process, as was also the case with the Carnevale and Springfield schools in Providence. Midway through the construction process, media and government investigations revealed the contamination history to the community and the general public, and a scandal arose [22, 53]. The elected school board, a political entity representing voters, worked to hold the school district administrators who had expedited the plan without public review accountable for their actions [53]. When the community's opinion was finally voiced, development ceased—but only after over $100 million had already been spent on the project [53].

We read only about the schools where a community has somehow discovered that the land beneath their school may be increasing their risk of health problems. However, low-income communities and communities of color have lower rates of mobilization and less civic support than more advantaged communities [53]. Therefore, we are less likely to know that such problems exist. This lack of empowerment, compounded by inequitable management of toxic exposures, as observed with the Springfield street schools in Providence and elsewhere, increases the pollution burden borne by such communities. Hence, the environmental and political injustices observed in school siting translate into health inequities.

In addition, health problems related to toxic exposures may take a long time to develop. Community members identified that an unusually high number of alumni of Beverly Hills High School, located in one of the wealthiest neighborhoods of Los Angeles, had developed cancer at young ages. Beverly Hills High School, it turned out, was sited on top of an oil field, and had been for decades [54]. However, because cancer is not an immediate reaction to environmental exposures—Beverly Hills alumni did not get diagnosed until at least 10 to15 years after attending the high school—it is harder to track and connect back to a specific source of exposure. The Beverly Hills High School case demonstrates that, although poor communities are more likely to be burdened with schools sited in unhealthy locations, no community is immune. With the long latency of many health problems, and the ubiquity of pollution, it may be difficult to identify the health risk of a particular toxic exposure—such as being exposed to pollution at school—but it is within our best interest as a society to reduce toxic exposures, especially among vulnerable populations.

More recently, contaminated schools in New Orleans post-Hurricane Katrina [1] demonstrated the extent to which issues of environmental, health, and educational equity overlap.

These case studies indicate that public health professionals focus on how vulnerable populations are exposed to toxic substances and consider how remediations and regulations may help improve health outcomes. Education policymakers are similarly people-oriented, but rather than a focus on health, they focus on investing in human capital, adopting an economic framework that considers school facilities as a requisite input for the "production" of student achievement.

WHY DO EDUCATION POLICYMAKERS CARE ABOUT THE PHYSICAL SCHOOL ENVIRONMENT?

Education policymakers are interested in investing in human capital—of both students and staff. Human capital, or the ability of each individual to contribute to his or her community's economic growth, implies a consequential emphasis on the economy and the workforce as a natural extension of successful investments in human capital, and compares school facilities to workplace environments. Improving the school physical environment benefits everyone who spends time at the school, in a number of ways, including increased student performance, better workplace environments, and additional jobs related to facility construction and management. Rather than the vast majority of education policies and programs that target a particular group served by the school system (enrichment classes for gifted and talented students, free and reduced-price lunch for low-income students, and union provisions for teachers and staff), infrastructure development policies benefit everyone learning or working at a school.

Investing in Human Capital of Students and Staff

A significant body of research exists linking educational facilities to improved student learning experience and improved staff working experience, and linking inadequately maintained school facilities to effects on teacher and student morale [46]. Some scholars have declared that the correlation between school facility quality and academic performance is well-established [46], while others conclude that relationship may not be conclusively causal [55]. (However, education research is rarely able to prove causality—for instance, we must also recall that teaching has not been conclusively linked to student achievement, and we can reasonably estimate that a connection exists [56].) Education level and student achievement is often used as an indicator of human capital [57], because student achievement is viewed as leading to increased economic capacity [58]. Investing in the infrastructure benefits everyone served by the school, rather than separate subpopulations [2]. Furthermore, education researchers, such as Greenwald et al. [59], tend to take on the perspective often espoused by economists: that the school setting can be considered to be an education production function, with school inputs including facilities and resources, and school outputs including student achievement and social and human capital.

The body of occupational and ergonomic research describing the effect of the workplace on the quality of work can be extrapolated to underscore the importance of maintaining a good working and learning environment for students and staff [7]. The age and condition of the facility (including temperature, light, ambiance, and noise) have been found to be associated with student performance [7], student achievement [60], and teacher morale [61]. One study compared students in the oldest and newest schools in a rural school district and found the students in the new building performing significantly better on reading and math tests, in addition to being in better health and having better attendance records [62]. One study of the effect of building quality on time spent learning revealed that over one-third of Virginia school districts had closed at least one school because of facility problems such as extreme heat or extreme cold over the course of two years [63]. At the same time, school districts are moving toward year-round schooling to reduce overcrowding or the need for portable classrooms [64]. The districts that need to implement year-round schools are often the most resource-poor, but they would need to invest in climate control infrastructure for their schools in order to make them functional at all times of year, thereby trading the problem of overcrowding for the problem of extreme indoor temperatures. Furthermore, inappropriate and/or insufficient space for classes is widespread and decreases the effectiveness of teaching [63]. Finally, facility-related problems, including allergies and injuries, caused students to be absent from school in 7 percent of Virginia districts [63].

Students are not the only ones affected by the quality of school facilities. Researchers have found that school facility quality has a larger effect on teacher satisfaction than do low salaries and contributes to a teacher's decision to quit [65, 66].

Investing in Labor

In addition to investing in students and staff, investing in physical infrastructure necessitates a major investment in labor to construct the infrastructure needed. Education policymakers' emphasis on labor may be because education and labor are often combined in the same legislative committee, as is the case in the U.S. Congress. As noted in the earlier analysis of letters of support for the 21st Century High-Performing Public School Facilities Act, one-third of the letters came from labor associations which would stand to benefit economically from increased investments in school construction. However, the benefits of improved school facilities on labor have been discussed almost entirely in the political arena rather than in the research literature. There are two possible explanations for this discrepancy: that the same legislative committee often addresses education and labor policy issues, and that the labor benefits associated with school facilities are not a primary motivation for building healthy schools. Regardless of the rationale, this component represents another way in which investing in school facilities leads to investment in human capital.

Education Adequacy and Education Excellence

Education policymakers define adequacy and excellence in terms of the quality of the "inputs" available at schools that lead to improved student achievement.

Education Adequacy

Adequacy can be defined in three ways: how inputs such as funding are used, what the process for determining the use of facilities is, and how outputs like student performance are improved [46]. The distinction between adequacy and equity is blurred, because major inequities imply that there is also gross inadequacy [67]. School finance adequacy cases offer two solutions to address inadequacy through resource infusion. One method, which requires fewer resources, raises schools to a higher standard as compared to their previous quality, but still keeps them below the top schools in the district or state. The other method requires additional resources to bring all schools on par with the top schools in the region [67].

A Tennessee state report finds that there is a positive relationship between "the adequacy of a school facility," or the condition of the classrooms and facilities, and academic achievement [7]. They note that a possible mechanism of action explaining this relationship is that school facility problems, like overheating classrooms, decrease the amount of time spent teaching and learning, the most important variable for student performance [7]. Overcrowded schools also have a significant effect on student achievement [45].

Students of color and limited-English-proficiency students are disproportionately likely to attend schools with concentrated poverty and overcrowding and/or deteriorating schools [68]. This compounds adequacy problems with social justice and equity concerns. The American Civil Liberties Union identified this special impact on students of color and low-income students when it filed the *Williams v. State of California* case in 2000, discussed in further detail below (see "A Tale of California Schools") [69].

Education Excellence

Policymakers have traditionally assumed that achieving minimum standards for school buildings would raise students to the point where their learning would be determined by the quality of the curriculum rather than the quality of physical environment, and indeed building quality continues to play a role in children's learning at all grade levels [7]. As a result, education policymakers work toward creating and maintaining excellent school environments to help improve student achievement. While education policy has primarily focused on maintaining minimum standards for school facilities, which have proved difficult enough to maintain, the introduction of the 21st Century High-Performing Public Schools Act signals that there is growing interest in educational excellence. The push for excellent facilities parallels the rise of standards-based reform policies that encourage academic excellence in the schools, just as the push for adequate facilities paralleled the educational equity movement.

A comprehensive study of all Wyoming public schools, carried out in the wake of increased interest in school finance adequacy lawsuits, found that school facilities do not impact student performance when controlling for other factors known to affect achievement, assuming that all children attend safe and healthy schools [70]. This study conflicts with the established research literature that school facility quality is associated with student performance, but agrees with anecdotal evidence like that stated by a parent advocate: "Transplanting an ineffective school from an old building to a new one is not going to change the quality of education. No one would be upset about school construction if students were already receiving a top-flight education" [71]. Perhaps this is because there is not a significant amount of variation in the quality of school buildings in Wyoming: The study found only 7 percent of school facilities to be inadequate in Wyoming, and no correlation between the socioeconomic status of students and the school building quality was found [70]. This lack of correlation implies that findings for Wyoming are not necessarily generalizable to all 50 states, because other studies in other states [22, 37] have demonstrated an association between socioeconomic status and school facility quality. That said, this finding also implies that school facility adequacy, not excellence, is the appropriate tactic to take in the realm of education policy, because there are no additional student achievement gains to be made with excellent school facilities.

A Tale of California Schools

As with public health concerns about school health, education policies regarding innovation and excellence in school facilities are only beginning, and there is no standard procedure yet. Plaintiffs in the *Williams v. State of California* case argued, on behalf of California schoolchildren, that some school facility conditions are inadequate for quality education to take place, driving educational inequities [68, 72, 73]. Community members were engaged in the preparation and litigation of the suit and the subsequent monitoring of the settlement. The suit, filed by the American Civil Liberties Union (ACLU), describes the heating and air conditioning insufficiencies, pest infestations, and poorly functioning plumbing that deprives students of the educational opportunities they deserve

[73]. *Williams*'s focus on resource allocation emphasized achieving adequacy for all and called for investments to address overcrowding and facility deterioration [73]. The *Williams* case called for all students to have the opportunity to learn the content material assessed by state standardized tests by ensuring access to textbooks, qualified teachers, and schools in good repair [69, 74]. By focusing on improved facilities and resources as a way to achieve these opportunities to learn, the *Williams* case implied that investing in adequate infrastructure was critical for investing in students' human capital.

While focused on achieving adequacy for all, the *Williams* case inherently emphasized working toward equity in education, and many civil rights groups united to support the ACLU [68, 74]. The movement for educational equity has been centered in the judicial branch of government, rather than the legislative branch, beginning with *Brown v. Board of Education*, and *Williams* follows in this model. ACLU attorneys described their rationale for a lawsuit: legislators had been unresponsive to their concerns [72].

This example demonstrates how policy advocacy and legal wrangling can be more effective when community members integrate school facility adequacy and civil rights equity rationales.

CONCLUSION

Numerous disciplines have contributed to our understanding of the effects of school facilities on students and the surrounding communities, and numerous groups have advocated on behalf of improved school facility policies. In addition to the quality of the school itself, both schools located closer to Toxic Release Inventory facilities and schools with higher respiratory health risks perform worse academically (as measured by the school-level Academic Performance Index score), in a study of Los Angeles public schools [51]. This finding links environment, health, and education and underscores the importance of addressing all three.

Environmental planners, public health professionals, and education policymakers are the primary people working on school facility research and policy, and the three fields approach the problem from different disciplinary lenses. Environmental planners offer a local perspective that emphasizes environmental justice and a regional perspective that considers the interaction between the school and the greater neighborhood toward community development. Public health professionals study toxic exposures and work to understand the effect of such exposures on vulnerable populations, including low-income children and children of color. Education policymakers consider how investments in school facilities translate into investments in human capital. Currently, the policy approach is divided by discipline, allowing each area to address school siting and school building policies from its particular area of expertise. These divisions mean that a number of government agencies may be involved in a particular project—or responsibility may be passed from one agency to another, with no one taking charge or having accountability. Our current regulatory system for school facility planning is almost non-existent and does not necessarily consider schools as requiring especial attention above and beyond other buildings that may not be serving particularly vulnerable populations like children. Future public policy could benefit from encouraging interdisciplinary policies and regulatory oversight of school facilities by understanding the common ground these three disciplines share. Lawsuits are another approach to address discriminatory policies and funding strategies that may contribute to inequitable school environments [1].

Underlying each discipline's work is a commitment to first achieving adequate school environments and, second, promoting excellent facilities. On a basic level, education policymakers have been addressing issues of educational adequacy and educational excellence for decades in other contexts, and environmental planners and public health professionals have considered issues of environmental justice and community-level disparities for years. By focusing on establishing what an adequate school environment is, and how all schools can reach adequacy in an equitable manner, environmental planners, public health professionals, and education policymakers will be able to effectively bridge their different disciplines to develop a more cohesive strategy for school siting and school building policy. Policymakers first need to develop minimum standards for school facilities and sites using evidence from each of the three fields to comprehensively define what an adequate school environment looks like. Community engagement is key to developing these definitions and implementing such school facility policies.

The case examples described in this chapter highlight low-income communities and communities of color advocating for adequate school environments as a way to work toward equity and justice, in comparison to wealthier schools and communities that often serve as beacons of excellence. While the three different disciplines have different names for this phenomenon—environmental justice, vulnerable populations, and civil rights—these communities share the same goals. Unfortunately, these same communities are often limited in their political power due to a legacy of disadvantage and disenfranchisement. The Providence case studies of environmental planning reveal that the school district voluntarily engaged with residents of a wealthier neighborhood working toward an environmentally excellent school and failed to consider community members' ideas and concerns regarding schools that were environmentally inadequate until mandated by a lawsuit settlement. This limitation makes it that much more important for school facility planning policies to emphasize meaningful community engagement in the research and policy decision-making process. The *Williams* lawsuit settlement led to increased community involvement in monitoring the quality of local schools in California. The settlement's website (www.decentschools.org) offers resources and routes of action for community members who act as local watchdogs as a way to empower those most affected. In addition to engaging communities in the democratic process, the examples of community-based research in public health and community-driven legal strategies in environmental planning and education indicate that more rigorous research can be developed and more effective policies can be created.

Recently, the EPA developed voluntary guidelines for school siting (available at http://www.epa.gov/schools/siting); the next step is to examine how they are taken up and implemented. The U.S. Green Building Council has also recently created a Center for Green Schools that is promoting the importance of school buildings [75].

However, regulations take time to develop and implement, and we must ensure that this is more than just a passing fad. As regulations requiring adequacy begin to be implemented, policymakers can begin to look toward creating inspirational models to encourage and challenge current conceptions of school facilities and instill the fundamental belief that exemplars are necessary for innovation. The LEED certification model of environmental excellence, and education policies that set both minimum standards for teacher quality and optional standards to recognize excellence, are examples of excellence movements in environmental planning and education policy. By combining tactics from the fields of environmental planning, public health, and education policy and aligning them to tackle issues of adequacy and excellence, we can more effectively address issues surrounding school siting and school facilities.

ACKNOWLEDGMENTS

The author gratefully acknowledges support from grant number 5 P42 ES013660-02 from the Superfund Research Program of the National Institute of Environmental Health Sciences, National Institute of Health, at Brown University and the Roselyn Lindheim Award at University of California Berkeley. Thanks to Laura Snyder, Phil Brown, and Laura Senier of Brown University for guidance and feedback throughout the development of this chapter, as well as to anonymous reviewers.

NOTES

1. A. K. Cohen and J. W. Schuchter, "Revitalizing Communities Together: The Shared Values, Goals, and Work of Education, Urban Planning, and Public Health," *Journal of Urban Health,* 90(2) (2013): 187-196. doi: 10.1007/s11524-012-9733-3.
2. S. E. Jones, R. Axelrad, and W. A. Wattingney, "Healthy and Safe School Environment, Part II, Physical School Environment: Results from the School Health Policies and Programs Study 2006," *Journal of School Health* 77 (2007): 544-556.
3. Howard Frumkin, "Introduction," in *Safe and Healthy School Environments*, eds. Howard Frumkin et al. (New York: Oxford University Press USA, 2006), 2-9.
4. J. M. Vincent, "Public Schools as Public Infrastructure: Roles for Planning Researchers," *Journal of Planning Education and Research* 25(4) (2006): 433-437.

5. S. E. Jones, N. D. Brener, and T. McManus, "Prevalence of School Policies, Programs, and Facilities that Promote a Healthy Physical School Environment," *American Journal of Public Health* 93 (2003): 1570-1575.
6. A. Cohen, "Achieving Healthy School Siting and Planning Policies: Understanding Shared Concerns of Environmental Planners, Public Health Professionals, and Educators," *New Solutions: A Journal of Environmental and Occupational Health Policy* 20(1) (2010): 49-72.
7. Ed Young et al., *Do K-12 School Facilities Affect Education Outcomes? Staff Information Report*, 2003.
8. U.S. House of Representatives, "21st Century High-Performing Public Schools Facilities Act, HR 3021 | Committee on Education and Labor," http://edlabor.house.gov/issues/schoolfacilitiesact.shtml (accessed September 16, 2008).
9. J. Vincent, "Public Schools as Public Infrastructure," *Journal of Planning Education and Research* 25(4) (2006): 433-437.
10. R. P. Lejano, B. Piazza, and D. Houston, "Rationality as Social Justice and the Spatial-Distributional Analysis of Risk," *Environment and Planning C: Government and Policy* 20(6) (2002): 871-888.
11. F. Violich, "The City Planning Process: A Framework for Community Education," *Annals of the American Academy of Political and Social Science* 302 (1955): 8-16.
12. People of Color Environmental Leadership Summit, *Principles of Environmental Justice*, 1991.
13. R. Bullard, P. Mohai, and R. Saha, "Toxic wastes and race at twenty: 1987-2007," *United Church of Christ* (2007).
14. R. A. Morello-Frosch, "Discrimination and the Political Economy of Environmental Inequality," *Environment and Planning C: Government and Policy* 20(4) (2002): 477-496.
15. USEPA, "Frequently Asked Questions–Environmental Justice." http://www.epa.gov/compliance/resources/faqs/ej/index.html (accessed October 21, 2008).
16. M. Greenberg et al., "Brownfield Redevelopment as a Smart Growth Option in the United States," *The Environmentalist* 21 (2001): 129-143.
17. J. L. Sack, "Scarcity of Property is Growing Obstacle to Building Schools," *Education Week* (2004).
18. J. S. Litt and T. A. Burke, "Uncovering the Historic Environmental Hazards of Urban Brownfields," *Journal of Urban Health* 79(4) (2002): 464-481.
19. F. Ellerbusch, J. Mack, and J. S. Shim, "Using the Triad Approach to Expedite the Acquisition of an Abbott District School Site," *Remediation Journal* 14(2) (2004): 85-105.
20. Childproofing Our Communities Campaign and the Center for Health, Environment, and Justice, *Building Safe Schools: Invisible Threats, Visible Actions*, December 2005.
21. P. B. Stretesky and M. J. Lynch, "Environmental Hazards and School Segregation in Hillsborough County, Florida, 1987-1999," *The Sociological Quarterly* 43(4) (2002): 553-573.
22. M. Pastor, Jr., J. L. Sadd, and R. Morello-Frosch, "Who's Minding the Kids? Pollution, Public Schools, and Environmental Justice in Los Angeles," *Social Science Quarterly* 83(1) (2002): 263-280.
23. M. Greenberg, "Should Housing Be Built on Former Brownfield Sites?," *American Journal of Public Health* 92(5) (2002): 703-705.

24. H. S. Baum, "Smart Growth and School Reform: What If We Talked about Race and Took Community Seriously?," *Journal of the American Planning Association* 70(1) (2004): 14-26.
25. Douglas S. Massey and Nancy A Denton, *American Apartheid: Segregation and the Making of the Underclass* (Cambridge, MA: Harvard University Press, 1993).
26. D. M. Crumbling et al., "Managing Uncertainty in Environmental Decisions," *Environmental Science & Technology* (2001): 405A-409A.
27. Deana M Crumbling, *Summary of the Triad Approach*, 2004.
28. K. Gowri, "Green Building Rating Systems: An Overview," *American Society of Heating, Refrigerating, and Air-Conditioning Engineers Journal* 46(11) (2004): 56-60.
29. G. C. Wedding and D. Crawford-Brown, "Measuring Site-Level Success in Brownfield Redevelopments: A Focus on Sustainability and Green Building," *Journal of Environmental Management* 85(2) (2007): 483-495.
30. Ashley Katz, "News Release: Schools Rapidly Turning Green Across America: Smart New Designs Boost Learning, Cut School Energy Bills and Provide Better Indoor Environments for Students and Teachers." http://www.usgbc.org/Docs/News/Green%20Schools%20Press%20Release_082708.pdf (accessed October 2, 2008).
31. USGBC, "Press release: USGBC Launches Nationwide Green Schools Effort: 'Fifty for Fifty' Initiative to Engage State Legislators in Every State to Develop Green Schools Caucuses." http://www.usgbc.org/News/PressReleaseDetails.aspx?ID=3811 (accessed October 2, 2008).
32. Patricia Jatczak, "School Facilities: High Performance School Buildings Program." http://www.k12.wa.us/SchFacilities/HighPerformanceSchoolBuildings.aspx (accessed October 2, 2008).
33. WSSPC, *Washington Sustainable Schools Protocol: Criteria for High Performance Schools*, 2006.
34. S. Fischbach, "Schools on Toxic Sites: An Environmental Injustice for School Children," *Human Rights Magazine* 32(4) (2005): 14-15.
35. ProvPlan, "Hartford." http://204.17.79.244/profiles/hfd_main.html (accessed October 14, 2008).
36. P. B. Lord, "New School on Polluted Site Energizes Environmental Coalition," *Providence Journal* (2008).
37. L. Senier, "Public Schools and Contaminated Land in Rhode Island: Using Superfund Basic Research Program Research Translation and Community Outreach to Foster Research and Advocacy," (2008).
38. ProvPlan, "Maps and Rankings: Economics." http://204.17.79.244/profiles/cw_mrecon.html (accessed October 9, 2008).
39. L. Borg, "'New' Nathan Bishop Aims to Bring Public Back to Public Schools," *Providence Journal* (2008).
40. L. Borg, "At Gregorian, A Sense of Anticipation," *Providence Journal* (2008).
41. S. van Zuylen-Wood, "Ceremony Marks New Life for Nathan Bishop," *Brown Daily Herald* (2008).
42. PPS, "PPS Announces 2007 Most Endangered Properties List." http://www.ppsri.org/?section=advocacy&page=20&submenu=Most%20Endangered%20Properties%20List. (accessed October 9, 2008).

43. Deborah L. McKoy, Jeffrey M. Vincent, and Ariel H. Birnbaum, "Trajectories of Opportunity for Young Men and Boys of Color: Built Environment and Place-making Strategies for Creating Equitable, Healthy, and Sustainable Communities," in *Changing Places: How Communities Will Improve the Health of Boys of Color*, eds. Christopher Edley, Jr. and Jorge Ruiz de Velasco (Berkeley, CA: University of California Press, 2010), 495-533.
44. R. Morello-Frosch, M. Pastor, and J. Sadd, "Integrating Environmental Justice and the Precautionary Principle in Research and Policy Making: The Case of Ambient Air Toxics Exposures and Health Risks among Schoolchildren in Los Angeles," *The Annals of the American Academy of Political and Social Science* 584(1) (2002): 47-68.
45. Robert Axelrad, "Indoor Air Quality," in *Safe and Healthy School Environments*, eds. Howard Frumkin et al. (New York: Oxford University Press, 2006), 2-9.
46. F. I. Ortiz, "Essential Learning Conditions for California Youth: Educational Facilities," *Teachers College Record* 106(10) (2004): 2015-2031.
47. G. A. Heath and M. J. Mendell, "Do Indoor Environments in Schools Influence Student Performance? A Review of the Literature," (2002).
48. Mark Schneider, "Facilities and Teaching: Teachers in Chicago and Washington DC Assess How Well School Buildings Support Teaching." http://www.21csf.org/csf-home/documents/Teacher_Survey/SCHOOL_FACS_AND_TEACHING.pdf. (accessed November 25, 2008).
49. W. Alarcon, G. Calvert, and J. Blondell, "Acute Illnesses Associated with Pesticide Exposure at Schools," *Journal of the American Medical Association* 294(4) (2005): 455-465.
50. R. S. Green et al., "Proximity of California Public Schools to Busy Roads," *Environmental Health Perspectives* 112(1) (2004): 61-66.
51. M. Pastor, Jr., J. L. Sadd, and R. Morello-Frosch, "Reading, Writing, and Toxics: Children's Health, Academic Performance, and Environmental Justice in Los Angeles," *Environment and Planning C: Government and Policy* 22(2) (2004): 271-290.
52. Joseph Schuchter, *Enabling Healthy Urban Planning in Northern Kentucky: The Case of School Siting* (Master of Community Planning thesis, University of Cincinnati, 2010).
53. S. Anderson, "The School That Wasn't: Politics and Pollution in LA," *The Nation* (2000): 32-36.
54. Joy Horowitz, *Parts per Million: The Poisoning of Beverly Hills High School* (New York: Penguin Group, Inc., 2007).
55. E. A. Hanushek, "Assessing the Effects of School Resources on Student Performance: An Update," *Educational Evaluation and Policy Analysis* 19(2) (1997): 141-164.
56. A. J. Wayne and P. Youngs, "Teacher Characteristics and Student Achievement Gains: A Review," *Review of Educational Research* 73(1) (2003): 89-122.
57. L. Wossmann, "Specifying Human Capital," *Journal of Economic Surveys* 17(3) (2003): 239-270.
58. J. O'Neill, "The Role of Human Capital in Earnings Differences between Black and White Men," *The Journal of Economic Perspectives* 4(4) (1990): 25-45.
59. R. Greenwald, L. V. Hedges, and R. D. Laine, "The Effect of School Resources on Student Achievement," *Review of Educational Research* 66(3) (1996): 361-396.

60. Linda Kay Lemasters, *A Synthesis of Studies Pertaining to Facilities, Student Achievement, and Student Behavior* (doctoral dissertation, Virginia Polytechnic Institute and State University, 1997).
61. G. I. Earthman and L. K. Lemasters, "Teacher Attitudes about Classroom Conditions," *Journal of Educational Administration* 47(3) (2009): 323-335.
62. J. H. Bowers and C. W. Burkett, "Relationship of Student Achievement and Characteristics in Two Selected School Facility Environmental Settings," (1987).
63. Daniel L. Duke and Jacqueline Griesdom, *Where Our Children Learn Matters: A Report on the Virginia School Facilities Impact Study*, 1998.
64. M. F. Orellana and B. Thorne, "Year-Round Schools and the Politics of Time," *Anthropology & Education Quarterly* 29(4) (1998): 446-472.
65. J. Buckley, M. Schneider, and Y. Shang, "Fix It and They Might Stay: School Facility Quality and Teacher Retention in Washington, DC," *The Teachers College Record* 107(5) (2005): 1107-1123.
66. S. Loeb, L. Darling-Hammond, and J. Luczak, "How Teaching Conditions Predict Teacher Turnover in California Schools," *Peabody Journal of Education* 80(3) (2005): 44-70.
67. Richard Briffault, "Adding Adequacy to Equity," in *School Money Trials: The Legal Pursuit of Educational Adequacy*, eds. Martin R. West and Paul E. Peterson (Washington, DC: Brookings Institution Press, 2007), 25-54.
68. J. Oakes, "Investigating the Claims in *Williams v. State of California*: An Unconstitutional Denial of Education's Basic Tools?," *Teachers College Record* 106(10) (2004): 1889-1906.
69. ACLU, *Williams v. California: The Statewide Impact of Two Years of Implementation*, 2007.
70. L. Picus, S. Marion, and N. Calvo, "Understanding the Relationship between Student Achievement and the Quality of Educational Facilities: Evidence from Wyoming," *Peabody Journal of Education* 80(3) (2005): 71-95.
71. W. Hu, "Despite Tight Economy, New Jersey Presses On With School Projects," *The New York Times* (2008): B4.
72. N. Asimov, "Landmark Deal Reached for State's Poor Schools: 1 Million Low-income Students to Get Equal Access to Good Facilities and Textbooks," *San Francisco Chronicle* (2004).
73. T. Timar, "Exploring the Limits of Entitlement: *Williams v. State of California*," *Peabody Journal of Education* 80(3) (2005): 126-153.
74. Jeannie Oakes, John Rogers, and Martin Lipton, *Learning Power: Organizing for Education and Justice* (New York: Teachers College Press, 2006).
75. L. Baker and H. Bernstein, "The Impact of School Buildings on Student Health and Performance: A Call for Research," *McGraw-Hill Research Foundation & USGBC Center for Green Schools* (2012): 1-35.

PART II

Organizing for Change

CHAPTER 6

"Serving Two Masters"— An Interview with School Teacher and Union Organizer Debra Askwith

Madeleine Kangsen Scammell and Ema Rodrigues

Debra Askwith is a teacher, union member, and environmental health and safety activist in the public schools of Springfield, Massachusetts. In the following interview, she talks about her experiences organizing around the right to public information as a teacher and a union member. Working with the assistance of lawyers, she has learned to maneuver in the hierarchy of city and school administrators as well as the city's department of education, finding allies and meeting resistance in a variety of places. She has worked on asbestos, mold, indoor air quality, infectious disease, and civil rights to protect all students and workers.

NS: Could you tell us where you are working and what you're working on these days?

ASKWITH: As a teacher in Springfield public schools for just over 20 years, I've been working at the elementary level and as a teacher of children with special needs. I am also a member of the Massachusetts Teachers Association (MTA) Environmental Health and Safety Committee. I was appointed co-chair about a year ago, and unfortunately as of today, I'm not on the committee because I'll be leaving this week for an internship with the National Education Association (NEA). I'll be attending four weeks of training, then a three-month field experience. Part of the conditions of accepting that internship was to give up any positions I held, but I'll be returning to the group as soon as possible.

NS: Please tell us a little about the work you've done with the MTA.
ASKWITH: I am a building representative as well as a representative for our local union, the Springfield Education Association. My work with them began when my local president said that the MTA committee was looking for someone; I joined and have really loved the things that they were working on, such as improving the working conditions and the learning environment for our students and our staff. I was really attracted to this work because it's an area that hasn't been addressed. We care about the test scores, but we don't realize how much health and safety can affect student performance as well. And even if it wasn't about test scores—it's about doing the right thing for people. So I joined the committee, and they sent me to the Tools for Schools Symposium conducted by the Environmental Protection Agency. I was so overwhelmed. I had just joined the committee; I knew so little. I was sitting at a table with someone from a facilities department in Rhode Island who asked, "What heating system do you have?" I said, "Oil." He said, "No, that's a fuel." I found out how much I didn't know—and how much I needed to know—before I could even begin to see if there were problems. I needed to educate myself about so much, especially issues around heating, ventilation, and air conditioning.

So it was just an eye-opener to how much more I had to learn. Fortunately, I have Chuck Levenstein and other committee members to help. It is a small, but an extremely hard-working and dedicated group of people. About six to eight of us are always present; others attend when their schedules permit.

NS: Can you tell us, what did he mean by heating? Do you have a furnace or boiler?
ASKWITH: Yes, if it's hot air, forced hot air, radiant heat, steam. I have a thermostat here, and I get a gas bill, and that's about all I know. At home I have forced hot air, and I found out that, at my school, it is radiant heat: the oil heats the water, and the hot water goes through the pipes.

I went to Tools for Schools, came back fired up about making some changes in our schools, and found it so difficult to do so. Getting people to come to a meeting to join our Springfield Education Association team was really, really difficult. One of the things I wanted to do, because I found out I know so little about our system, was to invite the head of facilities, Patrick Sullivan, to a meeting. I was so impressed with his care and concern, his enthusiasm, and his openness to work with us. And they had already begun a lot of good work in schools.

I suggested that they go to the Tools for Schools Symposium the following year. My local president said if I could convince the mayor to send one of them, he would pay my way—I'll do anything for a free trip! I wrote the most convincing letter I could to our then-mayor, and he not only sent Patrick Sullivan, but he also sent three other top people in the facilities department. At that point, I had also joined the Pioneer Valley Asthma Coalition school subcommittee, known as PVAC; Kathleen Szegda, the coordinator, was amazing. She was able to get money from the EPA to attend. So the four facilities leaders, myself, and Kathleen Szegda of PVAC went to D.C. together to attend Tools for Schools.

We started networking and, before we even left D.C., made plans to meet back in Springfield. That's where we started getting some resistance. I've been at my current school for nine years, and we've had five different principals. There was a lot of turmoil. And when we got back, the head of facilities—this person was in charge of all the public buildings in the City of Springfield—said, "We'll have the first meeting at your school, Debbie, so it'll be easier for you right after school. You can get started, and you won't have to travel." My then-principal said I needed a permit to have a meeting at the school. [But if] anything, the building facilities guy, who was holding the meeting, can come in here anytime he wants. So we met, but our principal was very suspicious, even though we're here to improve the school.

After that meeting, the Pioneer Valley Asthma Coalition coordinator introduced Patrick Sullivan to a woman who was formerly with MassCOSH. They hired her and started the Springfield Environmental Initiative. The Initiative is a group of concerned people from the school department, the union, the city's facilities team, and other like-minded groups such as the Pioneer Valley Asthma Coalition. All work to improve indoor air quality. They have been doing a lot of wonderful things. I've had less of a role because they tend to meet during school hours, and, unfortunately, I cannot leave work to attend the meetings.

NS: What was your background in terms of environmental health and safety, occupational health and safety, before Tools for Schools? Had you been thinking about these issues?

ASKWITH: I started out as a biology major at the University of Miami in the '70s with the hope of either going into marine biology or becoming a physician, but I found out that I wasn't as smart as I thought I was. After doing horribly my freshman year, I changed fields and decided to pursue a career as a forest ranger. In the '70s, careers in environmental education or environmental jobs weren't as prevalent as they are today. In 1979, I was employed by a film processing plant called Dynacolor, a subsidiary of the 3M Corporation. They processed slides, movies, and prints for a variety of accounts—supermarkets, drug stores, chain stores, and other film processors who outsourced some of their work. I worked the third shift as a "twin checker," removing the film from the customer's bag, putting a matching numbered sticker on the bag and the film, then separating them for processing.

One of our accounts was from Seabrook, New Hampshire. On each of the customer's bags from Seabrook I'd write, "No Nukes!" Someone took offense and complained to the company. My supervisor told the crew that they didn't know who was responsible for writing on the bags, but the practice needed to stop. That was my first radical action, but the environment has always been my interest. As a young girl, I read Rachel Carson. When I was 12, I read every

Jacques Cousteau book. So I was always concerned about our environment but never did anything, never pursued it, didn't have any studies in it, so it's all fairly new to me.

NS: That's great, even though it's always a transition to realize that your environment might not be the forest or ocean you'd imagined, but rather a building that was constructed in the '50s.

ASKWITH: Social justice issues also really get me motivated. A teacher at our school was paralyzed in a car accident several years ago. She came back to work—fortunately our school is all on one level—in her regular room that first year. Well, the following year, they changed her location to a classroom that had only one accessible exit for her. The second exit had a step that she couldn't negotiate with her wheelchair.

She expressed her concern that if her only exit was blocked, she wouldn't have a way to leave the building. [She was told] that if it didn't have anything to do with MCAS scores, [the school] didn't want to hear it. When she told me that story, I was blown away. Then I told her I'm on the Health and Safety Committee and needed to say something. I couldn't listen to that story and not say anything. She begged me not to because she was afraid of losing her job. Here's a woman, a wonderful teacher, a fantastic person, whose life was radically changed, yet afraid to speak up for herself out of fear of losing her job.

When I went to Tools for Schools, I met a UniServ Director from, I believe, either Oregon or Washington. When I told him this story he said, you have to speak up. He strongly encouraged me to be an advocate for the safety of the teacher in a wheelchair. When I returned to Massachusetts, I e-mailed . . . that this teacher needed a second exit; it took a while, but six months later, a ramp was put on the second exit so the teacher would have two ways to leave the building. When someone's safety is compromised, but that person is hesitant to speak up for fear of losing a job—it's just wrong.

NS: What is UniServ?

ASKWITH: A UniServ Director is employed by a state affiliate of the National Education Association. In our state, the Massachusetts Teachers Association is the affiliate, serving several local associations, such as the Springfield Education Association. UniServ Directors are involved in negotiations, alternative dispute resolutions, education, and, in some states, recruitment of members. In summary, UniServ Directors serve as advocates for their members.

NS: As part of a national?

ASKWITH: Yes, MTA is part of the NEA, so that they are all tied; of course, the higher up you go, the more power and resources you have. The local associations don't have lawyers, but the MTA does. So when it comes especially to legal matters we have to defer; the locals defer to the state union.

NS: Have you had to defer to the legal assistance of the MTA?

ASKWITH: Not for Health and Safety, so far. It has come close, however. They are very choosy about which cases they take up. They feel that a lot of things can be resolved at the local level. As far as environmental health and safety . . . Sarah Gibson, an attorney who formerly worked for the MTA, is a member of our committee and provides good insight into the things she has done for health and safety on a legal basis. She has represented certain school districts. She is amazing. She is my hero because she's so knowledgeable. I've learned a lot from her, and she has helped me word things to be more effective. For example, to get a better response when I'm seeking information, I'll ask Sarah if I am entitled to that information. Then she will explain that under Mass general law . . . blah, blah, blah, and I'll put that information in my letter. I look at the language she uses when she's requesting information and model mine after hers, so she's been an absolute godsend to our committee. She does this all for free. [Sarah has been hired by the MTA for specific cases, but she serves on the committee pro bono.]

NS: What are some examples of information you were seeking?

ASKWITH: After the wheelchair incident, I faced another issue. We had [an administrator] who required all staff members to display certain documents in our classroom; one of the teachers, however, remarked that it was a violation of the fire code. The [administrator] said, in front of the entire staff, "I don't care about the laws, I'm in charge of this building, not the fire department, I say put them up." That really got under my skin. For about a month, however, I didn't do anything.

Then, I heard a heart-wrenching story about a factory in Texas that, a few years back, had an explosion which killed workers. I just knew there must have been people at that factory who were aware of violations but chose not to speak up. Workers died. The people who knew about violations were just as guilty as the people who did not fix the violations. By being silent, I was going to be a part of the problem. Someone suggested that I make an anonymous phone call to report our school to the fire department. I called and gave my name, but they were nice in not using it. They visited several times. Eventually, they [imposed a fine] for noncompliance. We finally complied. It is nice to learn that you can do things anonymously. It is an action, and if someone's health is impacted positively, then that's a good thing.

Also, our committee has been working on an AHERA—Asbestos Hazard Emergency Response Act—regulation. They were talking about it; and, again, because I'm not knowledgeable in this field, I expressed the desire to see the report because Sarah [Gibson] was explaining the requirements that, according to the law, every three years they would have to re-inspect. I offered to check this out. I wanted to go back to my school, see about this, and learn about it.

So I asked to see our asbestos management plan. The principal replied, "What's that?" I explained that any school with asbestos has to have a management plan. She said she would look into it. About a week later, the principal located it. I examined the paperwork, and, in an effort to learn whether or not it was correct, I asked to make a copy so that I could bring it to our next meeting to learn more about it from Sarah and Chuck. The response was that she would have to check to determine if I was "entitled to a copy." I thought, well, I must be, but I decided not to say anything until I was sure of my right. I e-mailed Sarah to determine if I was entitled to a copy. "Definitely," she replied and gave me the public records law as a reference. But I was denied. When I inquired who denied me, I was given the names of two administrators. I sent them a letter. I didn't file a Freedom of Information Act request at that point, but I did contact them. At first they still would not give it to me. I contacted the deputy solicitor to find out, and she helped me in our city. Eventually I got the permission to copy the information that I was seeking, but it wouldn't have been possible if Sarah hadn't explained my rights to this information. I did more research on the computer, too, and found that the state law is actually a little better. I think it is chapter 66, and there's also another chapter 150e, that Sarah told me about. (I hope I'm getting the numbers correct.) It's about the right of unions to this information, so I hit them from all three sides. They took a little bit better notice then, because I had filed a complaint with the Office of Civil Rights (OCR) the previous year and had won. I filed a complaint on behalf of two of my students, and they prevailed. And I filed a second one and found out that I had prevailed on that one as well. I am not well-liked in my city—I can tell you that much. So they're very leery of giving Debbie any information these days.

NS: But it sounds like the deputy solicitor helped you out in one instance.
ASKWITH: She did. Yes, she was wonderful; she couldn't understand why I was not being given this information. In fact, I just pulled out the memo I had sent to one of the persons who denied me, and I wrote a second Massachusetts Public Record request. My original request was on November 19, 2008; a month later I still had not received a response. This is how I worded the letter:

> This is a request under the Massachusetts Public Records Law, Mass General Law Chapter 66, section 10. I've reviewed the documents contained in the AHERA folder located in the principal's office at Daniel B. Brunton Elementary School, and am requesting that I be provided a copy of any and all documents contained therein. This should include, but is not limited to, the following documents: 1) the original asbestos management plan, 2) all three-year re-inspection reports, and 3) annual notices sent to parents, employees, and employee organizations about A) the location of the asbestos management plan, and B) any abatement work done in the building.
>
> Separate from, and in addition to AHERA in Mass General Law Chapter 66, Section 10, they are public records and, as such, the Springfield Education Association and its members are entitled to these records under Mass General Law Chapter 150E. I've been informed by Darcia Milner that my

> request to make copies was denied by both of you. As you are aware, I must be provided with all the information I'm seeking within 10 days. If you cannot comply with my request, please provide an explanation in writing.
> Respectfully, Debra Askwith.

Now, that is not the wording of a teacher. So it is so wonderful to have someone like Sarah who can guide you and really help you know what your rights are. Most teachers don't realize they have a right to this information. Parents don't realize they have a right to this information. It is unbelievable. I eventually did get it, but it took over a month, and I shouldn't have had to wait that long. Now, the facilities department was more than happy to help me, so again it's something with our school department that is problematic.

NS: Do you have any theories that explain these problems?
ASKWITH: Whenever someone is so resistant, I wonder if they have something to hide. They don't want to own up to it. We're not out to punish anyone. We want to see what the problems are so that we can work on solutions together. We also have expertise they may not possess. The school department is not in the business of health and safety. In fact, one reason for these problems may be that anything they do for health and safety might divert funding for other projects. Or, perhaps, they don't believe there are any problems. If there were, but someone outside the administration (worse, our union) were to identify and deal with it, that would threaten their credibility. Just the same, I think they have something to hide. Why else would they not want to give up information? They're even more wary of my requests because I have been successful in finding their faults through the OCR. But again, if you have nothing to hide, what do you care? The laws still aren't being followed; they have not notified parents. In fact, a staff member came to me earlier this school year and said, "Gee, they used to have that thing about asbestos in the school, and I don't see it posted in the staff lounge anymore." I said that we're working on it in our committee, and I'd look into it more. That's when I learned our rights and responsibilities.

Last month, I distributed to our school nurses a workshop posting for nurses; I had written "FYI" on it as well as my name so they would know who gave it to them. The principal was outraged about my action. Imagine, I'm making our nurses aware of a paid summer workshop to improve their skills, and my principal is screaming at me, "If I want the nurses to know, I'll tell them about it!" As the building representative of the Springfield Education Association, I get my own copy of all postings and am allowed to do with it what I wish. I asked her—in writing—the reason for being ordered to stop this practice, but I never got a response. Some principals, however, are very receptive. We might want to focus on asking them why they are willing to step up to the plate.

NS: How has it been getting parents involved? Have you made a concerted effort?

ASKWITH: As an individual, I haven't put too much into getting the parents involved yet. That's something I'd like to work more on. Parents are involved through the parent-teacher organizations. We have worked at getting other organizations involved, such as the Pioneer Valley Asthma Coalition. They have been a wonderful resource. They've conducted education about asthma, are working with the environmental initiative to conduct education programs, and are providing help to pass needed legislation or changes to improve indoor air quality. But I personally haven't reached out that much to parents, and, I guess, that is an area I need to work on, although I don't even know where to begin.

NS: Right. That's OK; sounds like you've got your hands full.

ASKWITH: I have helped individual parents, especially the parents of one of the students that I filed an OCR complaint for. She was very ill this year; in fact we think she had the H1N1 virus. That was our latest problem that was not handled properly.

A principal said that [the flu] was no big deal, things have been blown out of proportion by the media. She also admonished teachers who wrote "fever" on the note we send to the nurse's office. She said, if you don't have a thermometer in your room, you don't know if they have a fever, so don't write that down. She also told staff there was no need for them to be tested. "It was not a big deal," she said. One of the teachers, the one who worked directly with this child, was sick, went to the doctor, and was out for seven days because she had a high fever.

Another student in that classroom became quite ill, went home, and her parents got a letter because she went out on a Tuesday. They didn't call to say why she was out, so they got a letter stating that she would not be promoted to the next grade because she was out sick too many times. So the parents sent the child back to school the following week still sick, and called me and said, "I didn't want to send her but they're not going to promote her, and we don't want her held back again." They can't hold the student back for that. This child has already been retained one other time; you can only do it once in the elementary level. This kid came to school extremely sick, and when the teacher sent her to the nurse, the parents were contacted. They didn't have a way of getting there, so the principal said to send her back to the classroom and made her sit in the classroom all day, sick as a dog, coughing, coughing, coughing. Shortly after that the paraprofessional who worked with her became sick and was hospitalized with double pneumonia. And they put this child back on a bus at the end of the day with 35 to 40 other children to go home, and she was coughing. They said the coughing was nonstop. They could have called the taxi. They could have called the minibus. They could have driven her in their own private car if the parents couldn't come. But the parents themselves were so afraid, and they don't know their rights.

NS: Where were the nurses on this? Have they been allies, and are they generally "in" with the teachers' unions?
ASKWITH: They have been. Our main nurse at our school is part-time now. We have people who rotate in, so it's hard to get things done. I approached the nurses, and they're interested in becoming a part of things, but they're not at our building on a regular basis. In other buildings they've become a part of it. In fact, when we went to the Tools for Schools in 2008, one of our school nurses came. The Pioneer Valley Asthma Coalition got funding to send one of our school nurses, and they have been a big part of it. They also were in on our meetings; the facilities team called in the nurses' supervisor, so she is part of that initiative as well. They've been definitely on board and are big allies.

The nurses have a different union. In some places, they're one and the same. In our city, we have different unions. The only way that affects us is that we can't fund them, unfortunately, to go to meetings so they have to get funding from their own union or from other sources. They've also arranged for asthma education in our schools from the nursing students at Elms College. They came in and did some outreach to our students in our schools, to all our students, not just the ones with asthma.

NS: Elms College?
ASKWITH: That's a private school in Chicopee, Massachusetts. I don't think the nursing supervisor for those students is part of the Pioneer Valley Asthma Coalition, but she may be aware of it. I'm not sure; she contacted me and asked if she could come to our school, because we're one of the priority schools. The Springfield facilities team chose three schools and made them our priority schools to start this program instead of trying to do everything all at once. We looked at the schools with the highest asthma rates and targeted them as part of the initiative; then as things progress, we'll go on to other schools.

NS: Is that the Springfield Environmental Initiative?
ASKWITH: Yes.

NS: Great. So you're focusing on asthma in these schools—and are you explicitly relating it to physical building facilities issues, is that it?
ASKWITH: It is hard to do a direct link since some of these kids' home environments may also be contributing to the problem, but we know, if their conditions aren't any better in school, that has to be a contributing factor. Think about the canaries in the coal mine—they may be a little bit more sensitive, but whatever is causing them problems is going to be a problem for students later on—for teachers with several health issues, too.

NS: And do they attribute those issues to the buildings?
ASKWITH: The teachers do, but then the administrators will say it has nothing to do with the building. They are kind of disregarded.

NS: What are the building issues you deal with? I hear about mold, and you mentioned the asbestos.

ASKWITH: Mold is one of the biggest ones. Mold, mildew, in some schools it's actually sewage that backs up. Cleaning is not thorough, and there have been some issues. A few years ago, our city went from having custodians to having a private cleaning company. A lot of issues have since cropped up because that company doesn't do as thorough a job; the city wants to save money, so they went with this private company. If you squawk and say classrooms or bathrooms aren't as clean as they had been, the city accuses us of being against non-union entities in our building. Instead of looking at the problem, they just want to shoot the messenger. We've had an issue ever since we got rid of our custodial staff on the second shift and have hired another company to come in and do our cleaning. There's a lot of turnover in that company. There's a lot of concern that they're not getting the job done right. In fact, the first year that they cleaned our building, one of our school committee members, who was a former paraprofessional in the school, was on the news saying that the buildings aren't as clean as they should be. She had toured several of them, and they started bashing her—saying that because she was a former union president she was mad because the unions are out, private sector is in. When I heard that on the news, I understood that may be true; I am sure she is upset that it is non-union, but the fact is the schools are not clean. In our faculty bathroom, we've had mold growing for two weeks on the top of the toilets. I asked a friend to take a picture of it to send to the school committee member, and I watched it grow. I learned about mold from Tools for Schools.

They explained how tiny fibers from torn toilet paper float in the air and land on porcelain; if those fibers become wet—for example, this particular bathroom had a little leak—mold will grow, because there's food for the mold. Mold was growing and growing for two weeks; obviously they were not cleaning.

You could have just swished a rag over it and eliminated it. It's amazing, it's so obvious, so simple to remedy, costs no money—it is part of their job, but it was not being done. There are so many simple remedies, and maybe there's something other than resistance against unions by administrators. Perhaps they think everything is going to cost money, and they don't recognize that some things can be fixed through better practices. When things are done right, money is saved in the long run, but they don't see those implications.

NS: When you talk about the city and the facilities management in public buildings, how do charter schools or private schools play into that?

ASKWITH: That's a good question, because there are two different types of charter schools; some are now part of our union, but some are not. We have been having a big debate about whether we should let the others join. Because they are public, I don't know. That is a real good question. I was shocked when I joined the committee to learn that OSHA [the Occupational Safety and Health Administration] does not apply to our public buildings in Massachusetts. Isn't that amazing? There are certain states [where] OSHA has no authority in public buildings, and Massachusetts is one of those states.

NS: Isn't there an effort in Massachusetts to get state employees covered?
ASKWITH: Yes. In fact, I was on the committee all of two weeks when I went to Boston to testify. [Massachusetts State Representative] Peter Koutoujian introduced legislation along with another person to have a law that offers protection that is similar to OSHA. The law wouldn't allow OSHA, but it would mimic what OSHA does, so that there wouldn't be that lack of coverage. When I tell people about it, they're like, "What do you mean? OSHA can't come into the school?" Well they can't. They have no authority in Massachusetts' schools.

Another good thing coming up for Springfield is we did get money from the school building authority recently that will hopefully improve indoor air quality. Our union advocated for and also got funding from the National Education Association to do parent involvement, to lower our dropout rates through parent involvement. And even though it's a different topic, once you get the parents involved in one thing, it's easier to keep them involved with other things as well.

NS: Would you tell us about your internship you are about to undertake?
ASKWITH: Yes, yes. I am excited and frightened at the same time. They call it boot camp, and it's beginning to sound like it. It is four weeks of intensive training; they told us to be prepared for ten-to 15-hour days.

NS: Where will you be?
ASKWITH: At the Bolger Conference Center in Potomac, Maryland, from July 10 to August 10, seven days a week. We will be learning all the things we'll need as a UniServ Director; about laws and regulations related to education and to unions, leadership skills, communication skills, contract negotiations, grievance procedures, and conflict management. We have gotten some great books to read; one of them is Rules for Radicals. So it is about activism as well. I've been told that you put your luggage in your room that first afternoon and work right into that night.

NS: What happened to the eight-hour work day?
ASKWITH: Oh, this is the union, cut us some slack. [Laughter.] I am thinking it will be a lot like the representative assembly for the National Educational Association each year. This year it was held in San Diego; it's a week-long event of meetings and long days. I actually enjoy them. It is so interesting; you don't realize you're there as long as you are. So I'm hoping this will be a lot like our annual meeting where I don't mind the 12-hour days. It really is fascinating.

NS: After August 10, you return for just a few days before you do your field work?
ASKWITH: Yes, you come back for seven to 10 days depending on where you're being sent. We won't know where we will be going until the end of our

training session. They try to look at your weaknesses and send you someplace that will help you overcome them. So if they find out that grievances are my weakness, they will find a state affiliation where they are currently doing a lot of work in that area, so I can get more experience and turn my weakness into a strength. They also try to put you in a situation that is quite different than the one you are accustomed to. So they wouldn't assign me in New England. They will put me in a different part of the country. We are required to dress nice, too. Come on, I am from Massachusetts! I can't wear my jeans? It is always funny to observe the regional differences. You go to the representative assembly at the NEA, and 10,000 educators are there; certain delegations wear the same outfit, which is really neat. Alaska, they all wear the same jacket with the big dipper on the back, which is on the state flag. California always has interesting shirts—200 delegates all dress alike. The Hawaiians all come wearing the same shirt. We have a denim shirt that says Mass Teachers Association.

NS: And how did you learn about your internship? Is this an opportunity that exists for others?
ASKWITH: Yes, it's annual. The *NEA Today* published a brief article about opportunities for women and minorities. I had to complete a 12-page application; that should have been a warning. I interviewed for two hours; they flew me to Washington for the interview, which was more like an interrogation. But I survived. At first I thought, I don't know if I'm going to take this, even if I get it, but it's just an opportunity I can't resist. It's a chance to grow, to become better however long I last—if they don't kick me out first. It's all expenses paid; they pay my salary while I'm away, my insurance premiums. They pay our living expenses. They give us a stipend for doing our laundry and incidentals that we will need. How can you say no to something like that? You can't, and whatever I learn is going to help me in other avenues of my life and my profession.

And I do want to go more in that direction. I still like the classroom, but I find so much of my time being taken up with advocating for students and staff. It's getting hard to serve two masters. I wish the MTA would hire a full-time health and safety person, because I would love to do it, but I don't have the knowledge or the skills. But I know people who do. I can put the "bug" in someone's ear. I really enjoy doing that. It does not seem like work to me.

NS: We have one more question about Boards of Health in Springfield and their role, if any, in addressing health and safety issues with the schools.
ASKWITH: I haven't dealt with them yet. I don't know how active they are. I have not heard much from them, even when we were doing pandemic flu training. That was another big concern of our committee. Bay State Medical Center did a wonderful seminar called "Ethical Dilemmas for Pandemic Flu," and I think someone from the Department of Public Health was there talking about utilizing the schools as health centers should that ever occur, and what schools would be

picked and why. I usually never have that conversation with our partners in the school; I think that's something that should have been addressed. It would be nice if there were more interagency committees. They all have something to offer; it's going to affect us if they're going to be closing schools. We need to be a part of that discussion on how that is going to happen. But I don't see a lot of networking with the different departments other than facilities, and that was because we, the teachers' union, invited them in. They were more than willing; they were happy to do it. Maybe something else we need to work on is reaching out to them as well.

NS: Thank you so much. Have a wonderful four weeks, and thanks for squeezing us in just before your departure.
ASKWITH: It's my honor.

Editor's Postscript: Debbie completed her internship in Alexandria, Louisiana.

CHAPTER 7

"We Can't Give Up, It's Too Important"— Health and Safety Stories from Canadian and U.S. Schools

Dorothy Wigmore

Schools are supposed to be places where children learn and thrive; not where they, teachers, and other staff get sick. The hazards are many, but recognition of those hazards is hard to come by in schools in Canada and the United States. The result can be an uphill fight for school-based organizations and unions. In this chapter, representatives of four such groups, two each from Canada and the United States, discuss the hazards and their effects. They have many—often unrecognized—successes and related lessons to share. These include taking comprehensive approaches, looking for broad sweeps and entrees, using building sciences and strategies of solid information, acting with respect and with persistence, including students and parents, going for green cleaners, and using participatory methods. The representatives of each group build on these to discuss what else needs to be done. The ideas are underpinned by the creativity, dedication, and persistence evident in their work to date.

Known endocrine disruptors, mutagens, carcinogens, and neurotoxicants are commonplace product ingredients, often used without attention to preventing harm or exposure. Biological substances, such as molds, contribute to indoor air quality problems. Tuberculosis, influenza, or other communicable diseases are almost always present. Sick people often are expected to work. Whether a nuisance or a serious issue, these chemical and biological hazards are a frequent source of discomfort and ill health in schools.

Growing use of computers and electronic procedures brings ergonomic problems and raises questions about electromagnetic radiation. Stressors are ubiquitous, ranging from physical and verbal violence, bullying, and harassment to having a lot of responsibilities with little or no control. Workload and expectations are high, but respect often is missing.

The hazards are many, but the dead bodies are few and far between. Most of those affected "just" get sick or hurt. They are part of a largely female workforce that frequently puts others' needs ahead of its own. Is this what we expect in schools? Is this the environment where we expect our children to flourish and learn and the staff to be healthy, helpful, and dedicated?

There is a growing movement to recognize and deal with school-based occupational and environmental health and safety hazards: That is the message from representatives of four organizations in Canada and the United States. Driven by concerns for the health of children and school-based staff, they are bringing these issues into the public light with a range of goals and using a variety of strategies. Their work offers examples of practical experiences, innovative strategies, and successes that often go unrecognized.

Interviews conducted in 2009 with these representatives focused on the following questions: What are school-based hazards, and why do they matter? How do school-based hazards compare with those in other workplaces? What solutions and strategies have been used to prevent or reduce harm from the hazards? What are the lessons for researchers and activists? What else needs to be done? Respondents included: Darryl Alexander, Health and Safety Program Director for the American Federation of Teachers (AFT) in Washington, DC; Mae Burrows, then Executive Director of Toxic Free Canada (TFC), formerly the Labour Environmental Alliance Society or LEAS in Vancouver, BC; Karen Robinson, President of Canadians for A Safe Learning Environment (CASLE) in Halifax, NS; and Tolle Graham, the Healthy Schools Coordinator with the Massachusetts Coalition for Occupational Safety and Health (MassCOSH), in Boston.

WHAT ARE THE HEALTH AND SAFETY ISSUES?

Many schools have the full gamut of hazards named above. "They are very complex industries with all sorts of hazards that are related to the work people do," says Alexander. The AFT's 1.4 million-plus members include teachers and paraprofessionals—bus drivers, teaching assistants/aides, security personnel, and administrative staff. "By and large, the hazards are not recognized. It was the same for health care and hospitals in the 1970s," Alexander says. Recognized or not, she has more than enough work on her plate these days. It includes H1N1 flu and tuberculosis (schools are the number one setting for community outbreaks in the United States), many indoor air issues, "green" cleaning products, high rates of work-related asthma,[1] ergonomics, and stress.

Toxic Free Canada's Mae Burrows has her own list of school-based hazards. The Vancouver-based alliance of environmental and labor groups concentrates on chemical hazards and preventing cancer in workplace and community settings. In schools, this includes preventing exposures to asbestos in the buildings; mercury in thermometers; and pesticides and cleaning products as well as chemicals found in labs, auto shops, and art rooms.[2] Their inspections also include "hot spots of dirty electricity"—how computer labs are configured and what protections are in place. Back-to-back arrangements create a really "hot" room while computers set along the walls reduce exposure to EMF (electromagnetic-frequency radiation), says Burrows.

At the opposite end of the country, Canadians for A Safe Learning Environment has tackled school-based health and safety issues by focusing on building science and the products and practices used in schools. Started in 1994 with a small group of Halifax teachers and parents whose children's health was affected by school conditions, they also pay most attention to chemical, biological, and communicable hazards.

The group of volunteers has worked on everything from carpets (there are almost none in Nova Scotia schools now), scent-free policies, and cleaning products to pesticides and low-emission building materials. "We partnered with the Occupational Health & Safety Division of the (provincial) Department of Labour right from the beginning. Around 1997, we added the Department of Education, and worked side by side on extremely positive things for Nova Scotia schools," says Karen Robinson. "We worked on not only improving the status of the cleaning, maintenance, and classroom products used in existing schools, but also the way renovations are done and the way schools are built." The group also works on acoustic health, playground safety, day lighting, and electromagnetic radiation.[3]

More than 1,000 kilometers to the south, the Massachusetts Committee on Occupational Safety and Health has had a Healthy Schools Initiative (HSI)[4] for about 10 years. The committee works in the Boston area, takes on state-wide

[1] Schools are one of the top three sectors reporting work-related asthma to the Massachusetts Department of Public Health.

[2] TFC's activities are described on its current website—www.tfc.ca—and its older site, www.leas.ca (from when it was called the Labour and Environmental Alliance Society). The "School Toxins Checklist" is at http://leas.ca/UserFiles/File/Toxic%20Free%20Schools%20Audit%20Checklist.doc.doc

[3] CASLE's website (www.casle.ca) provides a lot of information about its experiences, as well as documents it has produced or with which it is associated.

[4] The HSI, its activities, and documents are described on MassCOSH's website at http://www.masscosh.org/what-we-do/initiatives/healthy-schools-initiative

policy initiatives, coordinates the Massachusetts Healthy School Network, and is involved in national activities through the Coalition for Healthier Schools and the Childproofing our Communities Campaign with the Center for Health, Environment, and Justice in Falls Church, Virginia.

As the HSI coordinator, Graham describes what she sees and hears about as "layers of hazards." Many are related to design and maintenance of buildings—bad ventilation, materials that give off volatile organic compounds (VOCs), carpeting versus hard surfaces, molds, dirt, pests, and overuse of cleaners. Some are "traditional hazards that plague buildings, such as asbestos, lead in window frames and paints, and PCBs in window caulking. Other hazards are inherited when schools are built on contaminated sites," she says.

WHY ARE SCHOOL HAZARDS IMPORTANT?

All the women interviewed are emphatic that school-based health and safety and environmental hazards are important. Graham's response was typical:

> Short-term, because we always say teachers can't teach and kids can't learn if they can't breathe. Long-term, it's a workplace, for children and adults, and there are long-term consequences of being exposed to hazards in schools, hazards like asbestos, endocrine disruptor chemicals, off-gasses, building materials.

"It's also important because we do see cancer clusters, for example, in teaching and custodial populations," Burrows said. "We want to prevent cancer and take an approach about the timing of the dose (e.g., for neurotoxins and endocrine disruptors), especially for young children and teenagers, because of their critical developmental times."

WHAT'S DIFFERENT ABOUT SCHOOLS? WHAT'S THE SAME AS OTHER WORKPLACES?

Schools are workplaces, but are they different from other job settings? Yes and no, these women say. For example, location makes a difference. Canada's labor and occupational health and safety (OHS) laws treat school workers like others. Unions represent and bargain for all public-school-based employees in the country. Whatever their positions, they have the same health and safety rights to know about workplace hazards, participate in joint health and safety committees (except in Alberta, which does not require these committees), and the right to refuse work that is unhealthy or unsafe (the specifics depend on the province's law[5]).

[5] The Canadian Centre for Occupational Health and Safety has links to all the country's OHS laws at http://www.ccohs.ca/oshanswers/information/govt.html

In the United States, however, school-based workers may not have the right to organize or negotiate collectively. The federal Occupational Safety and Health Act (OSHA) applies only to public sector employees in 26 states; others have very limited OSHA coverage. U.S. OSHA laws do not include the right to refuse unsafe or unhealthy work, and few require joint committees.

Another difference between schools and other workplaces is that some of the problems in schools have no geographic or legal boundaries. "The biggest one is that we're dealing with the developing bodies of children," Robinson says. "From a health point of view, it's essential we get this right. It's important they graduate with their diplomas and their health intact. . . . It's the whole fabric of our future."

For Burrows, children's presence also is important in another way. "Kids have a sort of a second-hand exposure. It's the same in hospitals. Those who are second-hand-exposed think they do not have a right to participate in how the exposure is eliminated or mediated."

Robinson sees commonalities, too:

> There are exposures for employees. People that work in those environments have rights to demand substitutions for those exposures. Like those working in other kinds of caring professions, school staff members usually don't think of themselves very much as workers. So, often they don't have the same orientation to asserting their health and safety rights or asserting good health and safety practices. I've been on five joint health and safety committees. On each one, the teacher representatives must be reminded they are there to protect staff. They learn that they can protect children, too, by shielding themselves first and protecting the children second-hand.

There's also little helpful research in the sector, Alexander points out:

> Schools are supposed to be the safest places in our community, for our kids. With few exceptions, no one has thought to look at them in a really comprehensive fashion. No one wants to think about the hazards. Like the violence in schools, bus drivers get beat up at a very high rate. Special education teachers—parents beat them up and so do the kids; nobody looks at it as work-related.

Graham's experience with schools also is different from traditional COSH (community-based committees for occupational safety and health) work in the United States. "The labor-management health and safety model is not usually part of the school culture, especially if the unions are not really active. Even the Environmental Protection Agency's useful Tools for Schools Program has a hard time competing with the ever-increasing educational demands on teachers and administrators." (It emphasizes a multi-stakeholder team approach to improving schools' environmental conditions.) These kinds of differences between schools and other workplaces led HSI to work with community coalitions, health centers, parent-teacher associations, and asthma groups, as well as unions.[6] Graham notes, "It definitely broadens who we work with and changes some of the strategies, such as focusing more on environmental health rather than solely taking a hazards-based approach."

HOW DO THEY DO IT? WHAT ARE THE LESSONS?

The four organizations from two countries involve the full range of school staff, from bus drivers and maintenance workers to special education assistants and teachers. Three include parents in different ways; the AFT recognizes their importance but is not yet working frequently with them. All work in coalitions, with allies and/or in partnerships, and deal with building design and product uses. The union has ergonomics and work-related stressors high on its list of key issues, while the others recognize the importance of these hazards but have different mandates and/or specialties and experiences.

Comprehensive Approaches Work

A good example of HSI's strategies comes from its work about pests, such as mice, in Boston schools. In 2000, Massachusetts passed the Children and Family Protection Act. It requires schools to use integrated pest management (IPM) and to file their IPM plans. "There are templates to help, but no real enforcement, other help," Graham explains. "We found out most Boston schools hadn't filed a plan, and because we're focused on asthma, we knew it was a huge issue." Through the Boston Urban Asthma Coalition (BUAC), the HSI worked with parents of children with asthma who did a lot in their own homes. Dealing with asthma triggers in homes—particularly rodents—can be quite overwhelming for residents, says Graham, especially when costly interventions are required. When she brought BUAC's attention to the presence of mice, cockroaches, and rats in Boston public schools, the two organizations jointly challenged the school department at a public hearing about not obeying the law. "We rustled some feathers," says Graham. Eventually the department agreed to work with HSI on a Healthy Schools Task Force.

"The result was that we met lot of goals about maintaining schools properly," explains Graham. "Much about IPM is fixing leaky pipes, making sure windows close properly, fixing door sweeps to reduce cracks. We could talk about keeping buildings in good repair while explaining they couldn't use poisons anymore to kill the mice. We got schools to develop very good criteria for pest management contractors so everyone's at the same level."

[6]The Massachusetts Teachers Association (MTA), part of the National Education Association, does a lot of work with MassCOSH. See their respective websites for details.

The IPM project also made connections with families around their home and school environments and helped those involved better understand the many layers of roles and responsibilities involved. For example, the "blame game" points at kids' snacks or the clutter in elementary classes as the source of problems with mice, Graham says. "We've looked around and saw leaks under every door in the school and a leak in the sink under Ms. So-and-so's room, so we could talk about needing a more comprehensive look at IPM. We've broadened it to talk about breathing health and improving school maintenance."

Look for Broad Sweeps and Entrées

Looking for the broadest "hit" from a specific situation is a common HSI strategy. CASLE also goes for broad sweeps. Paying attention to building design, the group has had a huge effect in Nova Scotia and, to a lesser extent, across Canada. A 1997 meeting with provincial government departments that had a role in protecting children's health and safety at school was critical. "We gave examples about how the system was failing and invited them to discuss how to avoid kids slipping through the cracks. We credit that positive problem-solving approach, with respect, as the main reason that so much good has happened," Robinson says. That "good" includes CASLE's:

- Healthy Schools Design and Construction (2002) being integrated into the Design Requirements Manual for construction of all new public buildings in the province, including schools, hospitals and prisons;
- recommendations for full ventilation systems (i.e., 100% fresh air delivery) being adopted for all new public schools; and
- role that facilitated replacement of cleaning materials and art supplies containing toxic ingredients with healthier alternatives, reduced use of pesticides in and around schools, and reduced use of chromated copper arsenate (CCA) pressure-treated wood in playgrounds and new school construction.

Their entrée often is asthma and respiratory illnesses, "because that is something people can identify with quickly, the numbers affected are so great, and we can have a lot of spillover effects," Robinson says. Despite CASLE's close ties with the Environmental Health Association of Nova Scotia (EHANS), the group does not make environmental sensitivities or illness (EI) the main rationale for its arguments. "When we started, it wasn't seen as being real," she explained:

> The politics of improving buildings are very difficult. Those people get harmed in their workplace because others don't believe it's real, and employers are afraid of workers' comp issues. But they get the spin-off benefits of changes we recommend. Schools now do a lot to accommodate children with EI, but staff has a harder time. Salary insurance for sick teachers and workers comp cases still are not easy to win.

Use Building Sciences

From its experiences, CASLE developed a "new" approach to school-based hazards. "The old method was to complain, and then prove it. Health officials come in to test air or people and then say there's no proof the building is a problem or that people are sick because of it. They walk away and people are seen as second-class citizens for having complained, being sick." Now the provincial education department and CASLE focus on what is known about building science. They use clues from reported symptoms, health concerns, and building science to diagnose the problem. "When we work to make the building better, the health problems resolve." Functioning joint health and safety committees, sometimes called JOSH committees, also make a difference, Robinson says. "It's key for us to have the JOSH involved."

Solid Information, Respect, and Persistence are Key Strategies

CASLE's successes have refined its strategies. "Our three tools are solid information, respect for all those we work with (even those we perceive are hurting children, no one does that on purpose), and the third is persistence—we work in another way when we run up against walls."

Participatory Action Research Works

Involving members in activities is important for the teacher's union. "I'm very proud of work we did with Robin Gillespie in New Mexico with paraprofessionals who do special ed work with student handling, These paras have all kinds of ergonomic hazards," Alexander says.

She and Gillespie designed a program to give two days of training to about 24 special ed paras. "They went back and essentially became researchers." The AFT members collected surveys from co-workers in more than 15 school locations. Alexander and Gillespie used the results to write a report presented to the school district, with recommendations about next steps to improve ergonomic conditions for these workers.

"It was really powerful, and we plan to build on it in Albuquerque and, hopefully, across the United States. A Supreme Court decision says districts must provide adequate education for all children. We want to be sure that that 'adequate education' also includes safe, ergonomic environments for staff," says Alexander.

The union also has developed a unique six-session workshop about work-related stress that is being refined after two pilots. Union members are trained to deliver the sessions; they work with local leaders to identify six to 10 people in their school who might be interested in the topic. They use a learner-based popular education approach that integrates the participants' experiences with a framework of OHS principles, information about the hazard, and examples of how others have dealt with it. The result includes drawings of stress-free schools (Figure 1), body and workplace maps to make visible the symptoms and hazards, and recommendations to local union leaders about one or two priority stressors to tackle and strategies to go with them.[7]

Like the ergonomics project, it has taught Alexander a number of things:

> I learned that it's good working cooperatively with workers as partners for research and making plans for redesign of a workplace. You can't make a lot of assumptions that you know what's best for workers going into a situation where they live the exposures every day. I love participatory research; it's a powerful tool. It works very well hand-in-hand with basic training.[8]

Use Right-To-Know Laws

Cleaning products are becoming a common target for school OHS activities. For example, TFC staff worked with custodial staff and joint health and safety committees in several Vancouver-area school districts, encouraging them to look more critically at product material safety data sheets (MSDSs) required under the 1988 right-to-know law called the Workplace Hazardous Materials Information System (WHMIS). "Even with really good committees and really good districts, that wasn't being done in 2000," Burrows says. Using work with the provincial building authority, its CancerSmart Consumer Guide[9] and the Cleaners, Toxins and the Ecosystem Project,[10] TFC developed a list of chemicals that should and can be replaced, particularly in cleaning products. They use it with joint health and safety committees, parents' groups, students, and school boards.

"At the beginning, it was custodians taking the booklet [about cleaners] to their joint committee and asking them to go through products for these chemicals, saying 'We don't want to use them.' We learned that people didn't know what their exposures were," Burrows says. "They are very focused and committed to getting substitutions when they realised what their exposures were.

[7]The five-step framework, mapping instructions, and "solutions chart" are similar to materials the author published in a project for the Manitoba Workers' Compensation Board. *Seeing the Workplace with New Eyes: A Self-Help Guide for Workplace Safety and Health Committees and Workplace Safety and Health Representatives* can be found at http://www.wigmorising.ca or http://www.mgeu.ca/news-and-multimedia/news/read,article/95/seeing-the-workplace-with-new-eyes

[8]For other examples of participatory action research, see the special issue of *New Solutions,* 15:1 (2005) on the topic.

[9]The third edition of the 52-page booklet, featured on the CBC TV documentary "Chasing the Cancer Answer" is available on-line at http://leas.ca/CancerSmart-3-The-Consumer-Guide.htm

[10]For information about the project, a copy of the *Cleaners and Toxins Guide,* and other presentation materials, see http://leas.ca/Cleaners-and-Toxins.htm

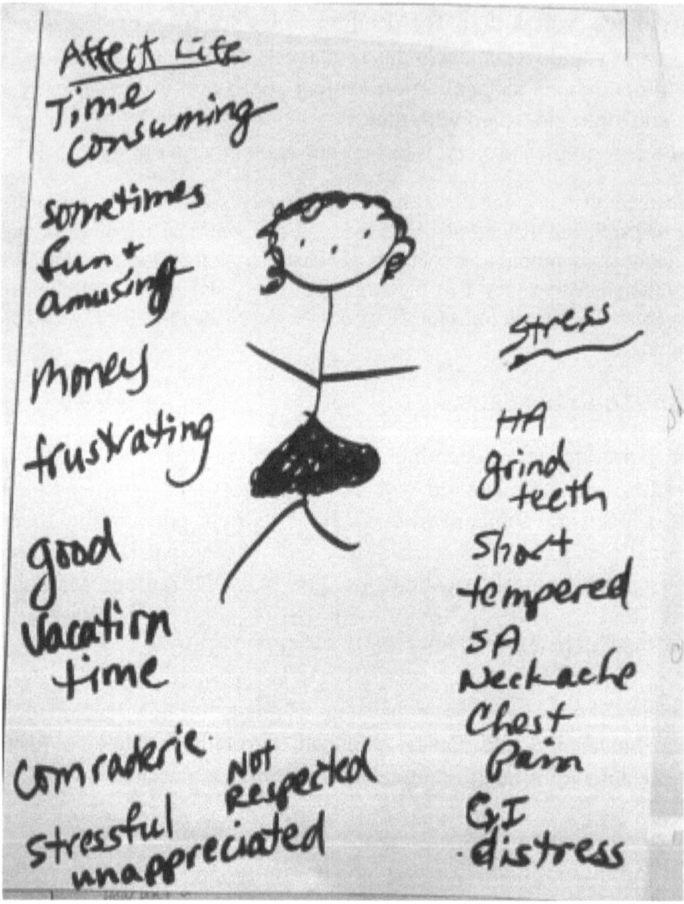

Figure 1. This was drawn by an AFT member at a pilot of the union's workshop, "Beyond Stress Management." Participants were asked to answer the question: How does stress affect your life? The list is typical of stressors that affect school-based workers.

They exert their rights under the law and force a substitution or elimination of something."

"We also learned that cost-comparative and efficient alternatives are available," Burrows adds. "In the districts, people would bring substances to the meetings, then purchasing would meet suppliers and say they had to find alternatives or lose the contract. We also taught people how to read the sheets and research the chemical so they could look for themselves."

Figure Out How to Include Students

But students often don't have a right to know.[11] That "birthed" TFC's students' environmental bill of rights. Following work with students and parents groups, the alliance also got a supportive resolution in 2006 from the British Columbia Confederation of Parent Advisory Councils, calling on school districts to look at all their chemical products for carcinogens, reproductive toxins, and endocrine disruptors and to replace them with non-toxic and "environmentally safe" products. The alliance developed a learning resource for teachers that has six modules designed to fit the BC Ministry of Education curriculum for several courses in grades 8 through 12.[12]

Push for "Green" Cleaners

While U.S. school employees may not have the same legal rights as Canadian workers, MassCOSH, the AFT, and others working in the field take a similar approach to push for certified "green" cleaners that do not contain asthmagens or other ingredients causing respiratory reactions. The "Cleaning for Healthy Schools Toolkit" is one example of their efforts. MassCOSH is leading campaigns for a "Safer Cleaning Program" in schools, hospitals, and state buildings, along with requirements that new schools and renovations use the healthiest building materials.

"Green cleaning seems to be a very good and effective approach to reducing chemical exposures for kids and custodial maintenance workers," Alexander says. "A lot of our members are proposing policy changes to their school districts for green cleaning and looking at it as a collective bargaining issue." It's part of the union's growing involvement in things "green." It joined the Blue-Green Alliance in July, 2009, shortly after publishing *Building Minds, Minding Buildings*.[13]

WHAT ELSE NEEDS TO BE DONE?

The successes are impressive but there still is much to do in both countries. Good policies and practices can be lost if they aren't integrated into the law and/or union contracts. The "players" need training about the hazards and building science. Differences between "green" and "healthy" must be reconciled. "To me, it's just such a huge topic and one that deserves a lot more research, a lot

[11] Section 13 of the Nova Scotia health and safety law says that people in the workplace must receive every precaution that is reasonable. The government Department of Occupational Health and Safety has interpreted this to include students. Manitoba's Workplace Safety and Health Act has similar provisions.

[12] For all these school-related documents, see http://leas.ca/Toxic-Free-Schools.htm

[13] See the document and related materials at http://www.aft.org/issues/healthsafety/buildingminds

more intervention research and better policies and regulations. I've done it for almost 20 years now and I feel like I've just scratched the surface," Alexander says. "We need national comprehensive standards about where schools are sited, how you build the school, and how you operate and maintain a school for health, safety, and security."

Robinson agrees. "People have learned and changed how they do things, but there is no regulation to force it on the school and departmental level. All we've gained can be put at risk." Standards about healthy buildings "also need to include ergonomics, stress reduction, lighting, etc. . . . We developed IAQ [indoor air quality] regs for Nova Scotia's public buildings in the late 1990s. They got watered down and watered down by government and industry and never passed. Maybe now's the time to try again."

To solidify already-advanced practices, by 2012, Robinson and CASLE started working with the Department of Education on a new project. Together, they are developing an on-line training module for school administrators and units to include in the curriculum. (CASLE's website already has the organization's *School administrator's guide to a healthy school.*) "There are so many potential issues over which administrators have control rather than building operators," Robinson says. "It also is becoming essential for citizens to finish school knowing how to make healthy choices for their lives, homes, and future work environments."

"I think we need to really work to figure out how to carve out that place for environmental health and safety as something that all schools have a system for managing. We talk about a health and safety management plan for industrial settings, but not in schools," says Graham. "We also need more support from the federal government. Citing guidelines would be great, as would strengthening green building standards, tying funds coming to states to green building standards. Otherwise, it's likely that if school boards are given money to renovate schools, they may do it the old crappy, unhealthy way. We want to make sure those standards are really in place."

But there is confusion between "green" and "healthy" buildings. "One of our challenges is meshing 'green' with 'healthy'," says CASLE's Robinson. "We're having a lot of success in Nova Scotia in educating green building folks about what's healthy. . . . We talk about the need to use the precautionary principle." By 2012, Robinson is encouraged by developments integrating green and healthy. For example, all new schools must have operable windows, and scent-free/chemical reduction programs in materials choices are still a priority. "It's still easy for companies to claim their products are 'green' if they do something as simple as use recycled materials in their containers," Robinson says. "The products can still contain questionable ingredients. Or, carpeting may become a more attractive option because of new low-emission, low-pile, modular 'green' carpets, when these features may not be enough. For health reasons, carpets must be as easy to clean, and be kept as clean, as hard surface floors.

This remains difficult to do inexpensively." Alexander also links "greenwashing" and standards. "Things can be 'green' because they're energy-efficient. . . . I definitely want energy-efficient buildings but I want them tied to a standard about healthy buildings."

Whether or not there are official standards or good practices, school staff need training. Administrators should be educated about the built environment "so that they can be good informed custodians of school buildings and buses and equipment," says Alexander. TFC wants more real-life, experienced-based training with MSDSs and inventories of toxic exposures in schools, so that there can be work about substitutes.

In the United States, taking school-related hazards seriously also means extending OSHA coverage to school-based workers. Alexander is not optimistic this will happen. "Some of my colleagues are patronizing, because we don't have dead bodies to show; we just have hurt bodies. I don't have big expectations of those running OSHA or those in Congress that these workers deserve OSHA coverage."

All these activities have a price, Robinson reflected. "It's been hard, hard work. Change takes hard work, and we were a part of that. It takes commitment. It takes networking and building credibility, being persistent and stubborn. Whatever we've contributed is added to what others have done. Everyone who's worked on making schools healthy places has sacrificed a lot, but it's worthwhile. We can't give up; it's too important." This statement echoes the words of the song "Rise as One," by Seattle-based Joe Jencks, which chronicles a successful school workers' strike:

> And we will never give up, we will never give in
> And we'll never, ever go away
> We will build a brand new future for our daughters and our sons
> We will work 'til all workers rise as one
>
> —Joe Jencks
> ©2002 Joe Jencks Turtle Bear Music[14]

[14] The full lyrics are available online at http://www/joejencks.com/index.php?page=songes

CHAPTER 8

New Jersey's Union-Centered Healthy Schools Work

Eileen Senn

Healthy schools work is taking place on the state level throughout the United States. Perhaps more than in other states, New Jersey healthy schools work has been union-centered. The New Jersey Education Association (NJEA) collaborated with the New Jersey Work Environment Council (WEC) to produce educational materials and training sessions, provide technical assistance to local education associations, and pursue policy objectives. Pressure from members, personal connections among individuals with experience in health and safety coalitions, progressive union leadership, financial commitment, and a change in focus from regulatory compliance to member organizing contributed to the genesis and success of the work. Others doing healthy schools work may discover new possibilities from the New Jersey experience.

NJEA is the largest union of school employees in New Jersey with over 200,000 active and retired members and hundreds of local associations representing teachers and education support professionals. The staff is organized into six divisions: Communications; Executive Office; Government Relations; Professional Development; Research and Economic Services; and UniServ, which assists and trains local affiliates in bargaining, contract enforcement, coalition building, and organizing. NJEA is the state affiliate of the National Education Association (NEA). NJEA has a local affiliate in every school district in New Jersey, almost all of them the legally recognized bargaining agent for that district's teachers. In many other districts, NJEA has one or more education support professionals such as secretary, bus driver, custodian, etc. An elected Delegate Assembly of 125 members makes NJEA policy, implemented by a 40-member Executive Committee. Policy recommendations come from NJEA's 40 standing and special committees, including two that deal with health and safety—Worksite Safety and Health and Working Conditions.

"Over the past seven years, the NJEA built a strong health and safety program that includes education, technical assistance, and policy work," stated President Joyce Powell when interviewed by the author via email on February 6, 2009. "We recognize the enormous benefits of health and safety organizing, including better working conditions, better staff and student performance, membership satisfaction, leadership development, and association visibility and credibility," she added.

Health and safety responsibilities were in Government Relations for many years due to the focus on Public Employees Occupational Safety and Health (PEOSH) regulatory compliance issues. NJEA officers transferred responsibility to UniServ in 2003, recognizing that health and safety was more of a servicing, bargaining, and organizing issue. At that time, Thomas Hardy, an organizing specialist, became the staff contact for health and safety. NJEA produced its first health and safety manual in 2001. The second edition in 2007 placed a much greater emphasis on activism. Local associations are encouraged to form health and safety committees, conduct on-site walk-through evaluations, survey members, assist injured workers, build coalitions, and use the media. UniServ supports locals in these endeavors. The current director of UniServ, Jim Geiger, was the staff contact for the Working Conditions Committee for many years and consequently is familiar with health and safety issues. The health and safety section of NJEA's Web site, www.njea.org/issues-and-political-action/health-and-safety was expanded and unlocked to make it available to nonmembers such as parents. Unlocking also permitted links to it from other Web sites such as WEC's site at www.njwec.org and Healthy School Facility Environments' site at www.state.nj.us/health/healthyschools.

WEC is a membership alliance of labor, environmental, and community organizations working for safe, secure jobs and a healthy, sustainable environment. WEC links workers, communities, and environmentalists through training, technical assistance, grassroots organizing and public policy campaigns to promote dialogue, collaboration, and joint action. Formed in 1986, WEC is the nation's oldest state labor/environmental (or "blue/green") coalition.

"WEC's interest in healthy schools work was sparked by the possibility for coalition-building between school staff, environmentalists, parents, and community groups," reflected Director Rick Engler when interviewed by the author via e-mail on February 6, 2009. "Many healthy school issues are also environmental issues, for example, school siting, pesticides, diesel exhaust, and green cleaning" Engler added.

WEC issued a report in 2000 on toxic chemicals near schools in Paterson and Clifton. [1] After a court-ordered infusion of funding for public school construction and renovation in poor districts, WEC saw the possibility of including construction unions in the coalition. WEC then issued a second report in 2002 that detailed the following policy proposals that set the focus for much of WEC's healthy schools work in subsequent years [2].

1. Ensure safe siting of schools.
2. Ensure healthy air for our children to breathe.
3. Ensure safety during construction and renovation.
4. Employ safety and health expertise at the school construction authority.
5. Ensure rapid response to imminent danger concerns.
6. Inspect new or renovated buildings before occupancy or reoccupancy.
7. Establish a Healthy Schools Advisory Council.

The partnership between WEC and NJEA came about through a combination of factors. Members active in the NJEA Delegate Assembly and health and safety committees, some personally affected by IAQ-related illness, were asking for more assistance from NJEA, which lacked internal technical expertise on health and safety issues. Two NJEA UniServ representatives, Norm Danzig and John Ropars, who knew each other and had health and safety experience with coalitions on occupational safety and health (COSH groups in New York and Philadelphia—NYCOSH and Philaposh), began discussions with WEC staff members Jim Young and Rick Engler about how the two organizations could collaborate on health and safety issues.

Because of the UniServ representatives' influence with internal leadership, NJEA arranged with WEC in 2002 for industrial hygiene technical assistance to be available to local associations via formal requests to the UniServ health and safety contact person. NJEA reimburses WEC at an hourly rate. NJEA Secretary-Treasurer Wendell Steinhauer, who serves on WEC's Executive Board, stated when interviewed by the author via e-mail on February 6, 2009, "The collaboration between NJEA and WEC has benefited both organizations. NJEA has learned so much about occupational and environmental issues from working with WEC."

EDUCATIONAL ACTIVITIES

The writing of educational articles on technical subjects was used to raise the level of awareness of the membership. In 1999, Norm Danzig, the UniServ representative with NYCOSH experience, wrote a series of seven NJEA health and safety factsheets by job title: security officers, secretaries, paraeducators, teachers, custodial and maintenance, food service, and bus drivers. In 2001, NJEA asked WEC to write a series of five factsheets by hazard (school renovations, indoor air quality, asbestos, violence, and bloodborne hazards) and two on tools for change (using PEOSH and health and safety committees).

After the factsheets were completed, the idea of a comprehensive health and safety manual was raised, and a committee formed to compile it consisting of the NJEA Communications Director, desktop publishing expert, the two UniServ representatives with COSH experience, three other UniServ representatives active in health and safety work, the WEC Director of Communications, and a

WEC industrial hygiene consultant. A manual was compiled which emphasized hazards, solutions, and Public Employees Occupational Safety and Health (PEOSH) standards. The UniServ director at that time, Vincent Giordano, noted that the manual had a lot of great information but didn't clearly tell locals how to use it.

This was rectified with the second edition of the manual in 2007, which stressed the following ten steps to effective health and safety programs that the NJEA now urges their locals to take.

1. Commit: Make membership health and safety a priority. Enlist the assistance of your UniServ field representative.
2. Organize: Form a local association health and safety committee. Establish a process to receive and respond to hazards and health problems.
3. Research: Examine district injury and illness logs. Review district health and safety procedures. See if the district complies with PEOSH requirements.
4. Document: Survey members. Conduct walk-through evaluations. Take photos or videos. Use checklists.
5. Educate: Use the *NJEA Health and Safety Manual*. Distribute NJEA factsheets. Hold training sessions. Show videos. Keep the membership informed and involved.
6. Assist: Assist sick and injured workers with treatment and compensation.
7. Solve: Prioritize problems and identify solutions. Pick winnable issues. Ask the district to implement solutions. Follow up to make sure changes are made.
8. Mobilize: Enlist the help of parents, students, community groups, elected officials, activist groups, and the media, etc.
9. Negotiate: Negotiate and enforce contract language on health and safety.
10. Use PEOSH: File PEOSH complaints when necessary. Know what is regulated and what is not. Participate in inspections.

Timely articles were used to maintain health and safety as a regular news item for members. Beginning in 2004, the author, a WEC industrial hygiene consultant, contributed over 45 articles to NJEA's membership newspaper, the *NJEA Reporter*, which reaches 200,000 teachers, school nurses, and other staff. In 2008-2009, articles covered topics including personal protective equipment, danger of damaged metal halide "R" bulbs, office equipment hazards, ensuring districts can deal with a chemical emergency, mercury, noise, lead in drinking water, power line radiation, art hazards, temporary classrooms, and engine exhaust indoors. Links to the articles are on the NJEA health and safety Web page.

Educational sessions have also been an integral part of building health and safety awareness. UniServ representatives Norm Danzig and John Ropars have been teaching health and safety seminars for local associations for many years. They also have been leading a workshop since 2003 at the NEA Health Information Network's (HIN) annual health and safety meeting. WEC industrial hygienists have also taught at the meeting, coordinated by NEA-HIN staffer Jennie Young, held in Washington, D.C. prior to the EPA IAQ Tools for Schools symposium, which is attended by 75 to 100 NEA affiliates each year. Danzig, Ropars, and others advocated for a full-day NJEA health and safety conference, and the first was held in 2002. WEC staff and volunteers taught many of the break out workshops and gave two presentations in the plenary session. The NJEA Worksite Safety and Health Committee, now chaired by Michael Wildermuth, a teacher at East Brunswick High School, has planned the annual conferences for the past several years. WEC has continued its involvement in the eight conferences held to date.

Health and safety training also takes place at various NJEA conferences, the annual NJEA convention, and at the local association level where it often focuses on how to form a successful health and safety committee. Thomas Hardy, UniServ health and safety contact person and organizing specialist, does much of the local association training. Hardy and the author have trained UniServ consultants, who assist UniServ representatives, in how to help locals form health and safety committees, use existing government agencies and regulations, and conduct walk-throughs of school facilities.

TECHNICAL ASSISTANCE

WEC industrial hygienists have addressed dozens of technical assistance requests from NJEA local associations. Many initial requests were to review and interpret industrial hygiene consultant reports, often on mold, paid for by school districts. Districts were telling local associations that the reports gave the schools a "clean bill of health" even when they did not. Another common request was to perform on-site walk-throughs of school facilities to identify problems and recommend solutions. WEC industrial hygienists Adrienne Markowitz and the author focused their evaluations on visual observations and staff interviews. Advice focused on what the locals should ask districts to do to address problems. By design, WEC did not perform IAQ sampling, for example, for mold or carbon dioxide. Instead, WEC used digital photos in their reports to illustrate problems. They have discouraged reliance on industrial hygiene sampling in favor of problem solving, believing that standards often either do not exist or are not geared toward the school setting, making them ineffectual if members of the school administration use the standards (or lack thereof) to resist improvements. The author has written about the pros and cons of industrial hygiene sampling in schools for the *NJEA Health and Safety Manual.*

DEVELOPMENT AND USE OF AN ADVISORY COMMITTEE

A Healthy Schools Ad Hoc Committee was convened by the Department of Health and Senior Services (DHSS) after former New Jersey Governor McGreevy's administration refused WEC's request to establish a similar, but more formal, advisory board by executive order. The committee provided a venue for advocates, the union, and others to work together. As WEC industrial hygiene consultant, the author led the group in quarterly meetings for almost five years from March 2004 to October 2008. Six state agencies with healthy schools responsibilities (the Schools Development Authority and the Departments of Education, Health, Labor, Community Affairs, and Environmental Protection) regularly sent representatives to the committee.

These individuals formed working relationships and learned of each other's activities concerning healthy schools. Advocates—including Thomas Hardy of the NJEA, Jane Nogaki of the New Jersey Environmental Federation (NJEF), and Joan Ponessa of the Education Law Center (ELC)—have had a venue for discussing school health and safety policy with these agencies. Healthy school advocates increased the agencies' awareness of the concerns of parents, school staff, and community and environmental groups on healthy school siting and design, indoor air quality, mold, pesticides, artificial turf, and a host of other issues.

The committee developed an agreement concerning which agencies could best address various kinds of complaints about school facilities. This agreement is reflected in guidance on whom to contact about what types of problems on both the WEC and Healthy School Facility Environments Web sites.

The Ad Hoc Committee helped WEC create the Healthy School Facility Environments Web site, hosted by the DHSS. The site contains key information about identifying, controlling, and preventing health and safety hazards in the state's more than 3,600 public and private school buildings. DHSS launched the site in April 2006. It functions as a gateway to online resources that help school staff, parents, students, administrators, architects, engineers, and contractors address environmental health issues in schools. With input from the Ad Hoc Committee, WEC prepared a May 2005 report, "Model School District Policies for Protection of Staff and Students during Construction and Renovation." The report was in response to numerous dust and noise problems with renovations in occupied schools. Updated in October 2007, it contains recommendations for school districts on maintenance of good indoor air quality and safe learning environments during school construction. The report can be found online at www.njwec.org/PDF/Reports/Model_Policies_healthy_schools_October2007 %20_ final.pdf

REGULATORY ADVOCACY

WEC was asked to assist the NJEA on legislation on temperature in schools after the 2005 NJEA Delegate Assembly recommended, "that legislation be drafted in collaboration with the Work Environment Council (WEC), which would require schools to be closed if temperatures in rooms rise above or fall below a certain temperature." WEC provided technical assistance on the content, frequently asked questions, and talking points for the legislation. A bill was introduced in the NJ Senate in 2006. WEC wrote articles for the February 2007 *NJEA Reporter* and the May 2009 *WEC at WORK* encouraging locals to lobby for the proposed legislation, which was re-introduced in the 2008 and 2009 legislative sessions. Bob Antonelli in NJEA Government Relations continues to track the legislation, which failed to come to a vote in the fall 2009 legislative session.

Lax enforcement of the PEOSH IAQ Standard was identified as a key problem for NJEA locals. WEC, NJEA, and the Communications Workers of America (CWA)—representing many New Jersey state, county, and municipal employees—worked in an IAQ sub-committee of the PEOSH Advisory Board. Among participants were Thomas Hardy and Penny Wells, a health and safety professional at Atlantic Cape Community College, who represented school employees on the PEOSH Advisory Board for many years. The unions won improved procedures for enforcing the PEOSH IAQ Standard. For the first time in the standard's 14-year history, a written protocol now exists for conducting agency walk-throughs, including a detailed inspection checklist. The checklist is online at www.state.nj.us/health/peosh/documents/iaqchecklist.pdf

WEC, NJEA, and others worked for amendments to the PEOSH IAQ Standard that would make the standard more enforceable and cover omitted issues. Recommendations from the IAQ sub-committee to strengthen the IAQ Standard were proposed in the NJ Register in 2006. WEC and NJEA testified at the public hearing in 2007 in favor of the proposed amendments. The amendments, which became effective in June 2007:

- Expand the definition of covered office building to include educational facilities thereby including them in the requirement to check and repair their heating, ventilation, and air conditioning systems when temperatures are out of the range of 68 to 79 degrees F.
- Define "Sick Building Syndrome" and makes it a trigger for employers to investigate the workplace.
- Assure the employer's "designated person" has the knowledge necessary to perform their duties under the standard.
- Require the employer to write a plan for how they will meet their obligations under the standard.
- Provide a 48-hour time frame for repair of water intrusion and cleanup of damp or wet materials.
- Require cleanup and airing out before re-occupancy after renovations or new construction.
- Make it clear that toxicity information for chemicals used in renovation or construction must be checked before selection, not just before use.

PEOSH has updated their educational materials on indoor air quality to reflect the changes. They are online at www.state.nj.us/health/peosh/iaq.shtml#forms

LOCAL ACTION

Better health and safety conditions in schools come about when local associations work to make it happen. The following examples from associations in Camden, East Orange, Passaic, Phillipsburg, and Pinelands Regional illustrate what is possible. In each case, the local association's UniServ field rep played a strong role. In addition, except in East Orange, WEC industrial hygiene consultant Adrienne Markowitz played a role, conducting walk-throughs, training health and safety committees, and providing expert testimony at arbitration.

Phillipsburg Organizes

When the Phillipsburg Education Association (PEA) faced serious problems with staff illness from mold in 31 portable classrooms at the high school and in the high school itself, PEA President Barbara English formed an association health and safety committee. It meets once a month with representation from all areas and buildings. "We have handed out surveys to our members to gather baseline information for each district facility. We expect that the school district's committee will work hand in hand with the association's committee," English said when interviewed by the author via e-mail in December 2008.

Health and safety Chair Marilyn Shober reports that a permanent solution—a new high school building—by the Schools Development Authority got underway in September 2009. The $174 million school had been delayed by lack of state funds for years. Meanwhile, sick staff members have been helped with Worker's Compensation claims and by obtaining some accommodations under the Americans with Disabilities Act (ADA).

Passaic Documents

The Education Association of Passaic's (EAP) Health and Safety Committee distributed a written survey to members in the district's 18 schools in 2007. The survey covered the status of safety and health conditions in all schools, including loose asbestos floor tiles, roof leaks, and garbage on school grounds. "Health and safety committees are being set up in each school," said EAP President Robin Holcombe when interviewed by the author via e-mail in December 2008. "Each committee is prioritizing the survey results to address them in a logical order." The administration has agreed to hold monthly meetings with the committee to deal with each problem. Asbestos floor tiles have already been removed and replaced.

Camden Educates

Members of the school staff in Camden face bullying problems in the district's 33 schools. Camden Education Association (CEA) President Ken McIntosh and health and safety committee chairs Dawn Colligan and Vires Simmons arranged for six building-level health and safety representatives to attend the 2008 NJEA Health and Safety Conference in New Brunswick. They attended workshops on gang culture, bullying and violence, using health and safety as an organizing tool, and mold and indoor air quality. These representatives then passed the information on to the monthly meeting of the 75-member CEA representative council for their use.

Pinelands Assists

The Pinelands Education Association (PEA) had several members with work-related illnesses believed to be from an improperly ventilated sewage digester and unvented copiers and laminators in the junior high school's media center. PEA President Pat Kloc, Vice President Jackie Stone, and Grievance Chair Joyce Weiss led the fight to get members' sick time and back pay restored. Arbitration resulted. Armed with documentation that linked the hazards to members' health, PEA won the restoration of more than 16 sick days to three staff members. District employees were also referred to occupational health physicians at the Occupational Health Clinic at UMDNJ in Piscataway.

East Orange Negotiates

The East Orange Education Association (EOEA) negotiated the following health and safety contract language: "The parties shall establish a permanent advisory committee whose purpose shall be to advise the Superintendent on matters concerning the maintenance of proper standards of health, safety, and security. The committee shall consist of four individuals appointed by the Association President and four individuals appointed by the Superintendent. The chair shall be selected by the committee members. The committee shall convene no fewer than five times during the year and will meet during working hours" [3].

EOEA President Jacqui Greadington appointed Vice President Clarence Osborne and representatives from several schools to the committee. The superintendent appointed the heads of security, maintenance, ventilation and the district's architect. "These people have the authority to create change," said Greadington when interviewed by the author via e-mail in December 2008. "Association and district representatives partner-up and walk room by room through designated buildings with a checklist, identifying any health, safety or security issues." It is then incumbent upon the district to address the issues discovered, she noted. At a subsequent meeting, timelines are established to address the issues discovered. Another walk-through is scheduled to ensure that remedial work has been completed.

UNION ACTION IN PATERSON

An early victory using the organizing model took place in Paterson School 6 where staff and students, reporting for the first day of school in September 2002, found themselves in the middle of a huge renovation project. The union forced the district to shut down the school and relocate staff and students for several months until all renovations were completed. Paterson Education Association President Peter Tirri and UniServ staff rep John Ropars conducted an immediate walk-through and arranged for WEC industrial hygiene consultant Ed Olmsted to do an emergency evaluation. Among the problems found were a boiler contaminated with asbestos being dismantled next to the cafeteria, classrooms littered with trashcans collecting water from ceiling leaks, contractors removing crumbling lead paint during a kindergarten class, and a 55-gallon drum labeled "hazardous materials" in the closet of another kindergarten class. The union successfully used media coverage to pressure the district to close the school.

More recently, violence by students against staff at JFK High School in Paterson led UniServ representatives Sasha Wolf and Richard Loccke to request a PEOSH inspection for the Paterson Education Association. After conducting a six-month investigation in 2008, PEOSH concluded that, although there were numerous substantiated instances of such violence, the district complied with existing New Jersey Department of Education standards for reporting incidents and conducting programs to support student development. NJEA has filed an appeal contesting PEOSH's failure to find violations.

Sasha Wolf and Thomas Hardy represent NJEA on a PEOSH Advisory Board union-management-agency sub-committee on violence convened in 2009. The subcommittee, which would not have come into being without strong NJEA advocacy on the issue, is exploring better ways for PEOSH to help public employers deal with workplace violence.

CONCLUSION

NJEA and WEC's collaboration has established a strong foundation for future healthy schools work in New Jersey. Hundreds of NJEA members, leaders, and staff have more awareness and knowledge of school health and safety problems and solutions. Many specific problems in individual schools have been resolved. Publications and Internet links are available on a large variety of specific healthy school problems. NJEA leadership has adopted and publicized ten steps for a successful local union health program. Explanations of various government agency roles and responsibilities have been publicized. Union efforts have strengthened the PEOSH IAQ Standard into a more useful resource tool. The remaining challenges and opportunities are expanding training and organizing work to win better policies. Although there remains an urgent need for better policies and better coordination of government efforts to achieve healthy schools, the DHSS has shut down the Ad Hoc Committee due to budget and staffing cuts. Achieving progress on persistent difficult statewide issues such as school siting, temperature, violence, and many others will require vigorous advocacy campaigns that include coalition building with parents, other public employee unions, environmental groups, and other healthy school advocates. Such coalitions would be powerful ways to build on the successes of past healthy schools work in New Jersey.

REFERENCES

1. New Jersey Work Environment Council. "Children at Risk, Toxic Chemicals near Schools in Paterson and Clifton, New Jersey, May 20, 2000." www.njwec.org/PDF/Reports/Children%20At%20Risk.pdf (accessed July 1, 2009).
2. New Jersey Work Environment Council. "Healthy Schools in New Jersey: Preventing Hazards to Students, School Employees, and Construction Workers, February 25, 2002." www.njwec.org/PDF/Reports/Healthy%20Schools%20in%20NJ.pdf (accessed July 1, 2009).
3. Collective Bargaining Agreement between the the East Orange Education Association and the East Orange New Jersey School District, 2003.

CHAPTER 9

Negotiating Indoor Air—Case Report on Negotiation of Teachers' Union, School Board on Air Contaminants

Sarah Gibson and Charles Levenstein

School districts increasingly understand the need for an indoor air quality plan, but may have difficulty in producing a plan that all necessary parties will accept. This article provides a case study of how one Massachusetts school district, after experiencing environmental problems in an elementary school, worked with parents and unions to develop a comprehensive indoor air quality plan.

The town of Westborough, Massachusetts is affluent, and its residents are over 88 percent Caucasian. Median house value in 2000 was $253,000. The housing stock is relatively young—this is a recently developed suburban community. Median household income in 2000 was $73,418, almost 50% higher than the state median of about $50,000. Of the population 25 years or older, 60 percent had college degrees, compared with 40 percent for the state. The 18,000-plus citizens of Westborough are served by six schools with 3,488 children, 272 teachers, and a 13:1 student to teacher ratio [1, 2].

In 1999, the town of Westborough faced an indoor air quality problem in one of its three elementary schools. The Hastings Elementary School was located near a swamp, which led to water infiltration problems on the ground floor of the building. In addition, ventilation intakes were located so that they drew exhaust into the school building from idling school buses and other vehicles. Forty percent of the staff complained about respiratory symptoms. Children had similar complaints. On the recommendation of a physician hired by the school district, the school was closed in May 2000, and its students and staff were redistributed among other schools in the district for the remainder of the school year while ventilation repairs were made.

The town spent $250,000 to replace the school's rooftop air handling units, adjust air pressure in the building, and remove carpeting in the school. The Hastings School re-opened in September of 2000. Health complaints from both students and staff decreased. Life at the school slowly settled back to normal.

There continued to be, however, considerable concern in the community. The regional office of the EPA had been involved in meetings about the problems at the Hastings school before it closed and had urged the school district to adopt the EPA's *Tools for Schools* program, the EPA's indoor air quality guidance took kit, or a similar indoor air quality management plan. Two members of an active parents' organization at Hastings, skeptical of the school district's ability to regulate itself, demanded that the school committee adopt an environmental monitoring and management program. They approached the School Committee with a request to implement *Tools for Schools*. They were turned down by a vote of three to two by the School Committee members. Not to be deterred, the parents organized a petition drive and returned to the Committee with over 500 signatures supporting a *Tools for Schools* program; again, they were turned down.

Faced with what they perceived to be an immovable obstacle to addressing environmental health issues in the schools, the parents' organization threw its support behind one of their active members who ran in the 2001 School Committee election. The election changed the composition of the School Committee. In the 2001-02 school year, the School Committee decided to implement some kind of indoor air quality plan.

Parents were not the only parties concerned about conditions at the Hastings School and the school district's long-term commitment to environmental health and safety. The Westborough Teachers Association (WTA), the union representing teachers and staff throughout the school district, had been part of the effort to pressure the School Committee to address the air quality problems at Hastings. The WTA urged the school system to address employee health problems—and insisted on health and safety language in the collective bargaining agreement. Initially, the WTA did not believe that the school district was taking complaints seriously and assumed that attention to indoor air quality problems would be short-lived.

FALSE START—FROM THE TOP DOWN

Invigorated by the election of new members focused on indoor air quality problems, the School Committee adopted an indoor air quality plan based on what it imagined was the best template available, one that had been developed by the Baldwin School District on Long Island, New York [3]. The School Committee looked to an existing plan in part because of its own uncertain support for implementing the EPA's *Tools for Schools* and, in part, because the idea of developing a plan of its own seemed entirely too daunting. The Committee was in the midst of contract negotiations with the WTA—and there was already considerable friction among the union, administrators, and the School Committee. The School Committee, therefore, delivered the news of its adoption of the Baldwin School District plan to the WTA in the fall of 2001.

The WTA, in its own words, "went ballistic," rigorously objecting to the plan's implementation. The Baldwin manual was not as comprehensive as the WTA wanted, but even worse, the union (correctly) perceived that it had not been consulted in the selection of or implementation of the Baldwin manual. The School Committee had viewed the Baldwin manual as merely a redraft of the EPA *Tools for Schools* classroom checklist, designed to make the checklists shorter and easier to use. The WTA viewed the manual as a re-write of *Tools for Schools* in a way that tried to put most of the blame for and effort to resolve indoor air quality in the schools on teachers. While the union may have been over-reacting (based on reasonable suspicions about the administration's commitment to addressing problems) and the School Committee may have felt that no good deed went unpunished, the WTA eventually took advantage of the School Committee's failure to consult with it and filed a demand to bargain over the plan. Both parties seized the demand to bargain as an opportunity to work together to review and redraft an indoor air quality plan.

FROM THE BOTTOM UP

Out of the conflict among parents, teachers, school administration, and School Committee, an IAQ Subcommittee of the School Committee was created in Spring 2002. The members included a School Committee member, the assistant superintendent, the facilities director, a district nurse, a school administrator, a teacher, a representative of the Massachusetts Teachers Association (MTA), and a parent representative. The WTA was drawn into the process of addressing problems by participation on the IAQ Subcommittee; the MTA sent an attorney who specialized in environmental issues. The parent representative was a certified public accountant with expertise in creating corporate best practices and improvement plans and was of huge benefit to the committee.

The IAQ Subcommittee's mission was to draft a practical indoor air quality monitoring and management plan which would include district-wide guidelines regarding procedures and communications and would establish school-based health and safety teams. The Subcommittee was to create an adoptable and adaptable template to be used in all the town's schools.

For the teachers, this negotiation process was, at least initially, a bumpy road. The union was still smarting over the initial draft and the perception of unilateral action. But even within the union, there were differences over what templates were best. Once the parties began meeting about a new negotiated draft of the indoor air quality manual, however, it became clear that everyone was determined to try to overlook past differences and make a good faith effort to produce a plan that everyone supported. All parties demonstrated flexibility—and perseverance. The drafting group made the decision to produce something that the teachers and the administration could live with for a year, then assess it in a year to see how well it was working.

Although the EPA's *Tools for Schools* served as an overall model, the drafting group often assessed what would work best in Westborough, and it individualized all aspects of the plan as much as necessary. All parties took on some of the work of drafting, and the group spent meetings in sometimes painstaking review of all components of the plan. Ultimately, Westborough's plan included commitments by the school district with regard to a variety of environmental health and safety issues; schedules for inspections by facilities personnel and building-based health and safety teams; forms for the transmission of inspection results to the facilities department and School Committee; and a method for the inclusion of maintenance and monitoring data in the school district's budgeting process. The manual can be downloaded from the district's Web site [4].

OUTCOME

In the Fall of 2002, the new program was implemented in Westborough's schools as a "work-in-progress." The WTA and School Committee jointly presented the negotiated plan to administrators and staff as something that both parties fully endorsed. The WTA participated in training sessions for the building health and safety teams at the beginning of the 2002-03 school year.

In 2003, Westborough received a *Tools for Schools* Excellence Award from the EPA for its indoor air quality management plan. In 2005, the School Committee renamed the IAQ subcommittee as the district-wide Facilities Committee and expanded its membership to include representatives from all six school buildings in order to improve communications between the Committee and schools. In 2006, Westborough received the EPA's *Tools for Schools* Sustained Excellence Award [5].

More important than the outside recognition and rewards, however, the new program heightened awareness of environmental issues in Westborough's schools. Awareness of health and safety has become ingrained in the school culture. Staff members have taken responsibility for their own spaces and common areas and are quick to notify facilities personnel of any problem; the facilities staff responds quickly and effectively to problems. Effective communication was critical. An important result was the establishment of a health and safety database which provides budgeting guidance for the school committee. Five years after the adoption of Westborough's plan, participation by all parties is as robust as when the plan first went into effect, and the plan has been fully implemented in all schools in the district.

Ultimately, the result of labor/management/community collaboration in Westborough was the establishment of an operative policy that may pave the way for other communities:

> *The Westborough Public Schools is committed to providing a healthy environment for its staff and students. To these ends, the Westborough Public Schools will:*
>
> - *Implement a rigorous inspection and preventative maintenance program.*
> - *Provide effective communications between central administration, school administration, staff, students and parents relevant to this manual, investigations conducted and remediation efforts implemented.*
> - *Maintain all building systems and structural elements in good repair.*
> - *Involve building occupants in all decisions that affect their health and safety.*
> - *Investigate building occupant IAQ complaints in a timely fashion.*
> - *Comply with recommended practices regarding IAQ and the condition, maintenance and operation of its school buildings.*
> - *Establish school-based Health and Safety teams to implement this program at the school level.*

LESSONS LEARNED

Many lessons were learned in the creation of Westborough's indoor air quality plan. Perhaps most important was the understanding that a school environmental plan or program could not be "top down": Its development must engage the people on whose participation the plan's implementation depended. The drafting parties in Westborough learned to view objections and obstacles not only simply as something to be overcome, but also as opportunities for careful listening and for gathering the information that complaints or questions conveyed. The development of the indoor air quality plan was complicated by the fact that a school environment involves learning—and working—conditions, and all of those concerns had to be addressed. The drafting group learned that it could not shy away from thorny issues and had to keep reworking the plan until problems were adequately dealt with. Finally, Westborough learned about the importance of record keeping. The future of maintenance and monitoring in Westborough would be built on an understanding of what had happened in the past.

REFERENCES

1. http://en.wikipedia.org/wiki/Westborough,_Massachusetts, accessed March 16, 2009.
2. http://www.publicschoolreview.com/town_schools/stateid/MA/townid/7634, accessed March 16, 2009.
3. Baldwin Union Free School District. *Indoor Air Quality Manual* (Baldwin, New York: Baldwin Union Free School District, Sept. 1999). http://www.emsc.nysed.gov/facplan/articles/IAQManual.pdf. This booklet identifies ways to improve a school's indoor air quality and discusses alternative methods for managing this issue. It includes sources and prevention, training of staff, renovation and repair, painting procedures, animals in classrooms, barrier matting, vacuum cleaners, IPM, chemical hygiene program, univents, IAQ flow chart, board policy, administrative procedures, and report forms.
4. Westborough Public Schools at http://westborough.ma.schoolwebpages.com/education/components/scrapbook/default.php?section-1, accessed March 16, 2009.
5. U.S. Environmental Protection Agency, "*IAQ Tools for Schools Program, 2006 Excellence Awards Winners*," news release at http://www.epa.gov/iaq/schools/tfsawards2006.htm#Westborough_School_District, accessed March 16, 2009.

CHAPTER 10

School Custodians and Green Cleaners: Labor-Environment Coalitions and Toxics Reduction

Laura Senier, Brian Mayer, Phil Brown, and Rachel Morello-Frosch

In the fall of 2003, the Boston Urban Asthma Coalition (BUAC) and the Massachusetts Committee on Occupational Safety and Health (MassCOSH) launched the Green Cleaners Project, a coalition of organizations, including labor unions and school administrators, to address well-documented problems of environmental quality in Boston schools. Coalition participants wanted to ensure that discussions about environmental health problems in Boston schools and their remediation would include the broadest possible array of stakeholders, including parents, teachers and other school employees, school administrators, and community health advocates. Despite the expensive and capital-intensive nature of solutions to many of the environmental health problems documented in the schools, the coalition quickly won a major victory on one component of its short-term agenda: the replacement of common cleaning products with less toxic "green" alternatives.

The Green Cleaners Project has brought Boston in step with a growing national movement to improve environmental health in schools. Over the past decade, community groups and advocates have pointed to increasing rates among schoolchildren of chronic illnesses (such as asthma and diabetes) and learning disabilities, many of which may be caused by or exacerbated by environmental conditions. The movement has also protested inappropriate school siting, both for new construction and for existing facilities that have been sited on toxic landfills or brownfields, or adjacent to polluting facilities. Movement activists have also sought to influence the design of new schools by pressing for the adoption of energy-efficient materials and green building standards [1].

Boston's experience in school health advocacy projects has also, however, exemplified many of the challenges in uniting participants in two important social movements: organized labor and the environmental movement. Alliances between labor unions and environmental organizations, or "blue-green" alliances, have historically faced formidable obstacles, typically articulated as a class divide that forces union workers to choose between job security and environmental reforms [2, 3]. Pressured by management to side with the political interests of industry, union workers have often found themselves in opposition to the agenda of the environmental movement. Yet despite recent high-profile examples of cases in which the pursuit of goals on the environmental agenda has threatened labor union jobs, there is a much older tradition of labor unionists and activists working together with environmental health activists, such as occupational health specialists and sanitarians, on issues of importance to both constituencies [3, 4].

The member organizations in the Green Cleaners Project are also participants in a regional blue-green coalition known as the Alliance for a Healthy Tomorrow (the Alliance), a larger initiative to foster relationships and political partnerships between labor unions and environmental organizations in Massachusetts. In this respect, the Green Cleaners Project operates within a tradition of cross-movement cooperation and shows the importance of health concerns as a common issue that, in favorable circumstances, may draw additional partners into the blue-green coalition and motivate both groups to work toward a common goal.

Our analysis focuses on two factors that led to the early success of this coalition and may assure its long-term stability, and which may suggest pathways and strategies to organizing diverse stakeholders around occupational and environmental health in a range of similar circumstances. We show, first, how the Green Cleaners Project team assembled a diverse group of stakeholders and, second, how they maintained cohesion by merging concerns about a high-profile school health issue with a precautionary approach to managing school environmental quality. Invocation of the precautionary principle facilitated the construction of a frame that represented the individual and common interests of all stakeholders.

Although numerous other blue-green alliances have sprung up across the country in the past decade [2, 5, 6], the Green Cleaners Project is unique in securing the cooperation and involvement of environmental and community health advocates, labor unions, and school administrators, and thus it displays a level of organizational complexity that blue-green coalitions frequently lack. We highlight the role of "bridge builders" who negotiated a shared understanding between the stakeholders about the importance of eliminating toxic cleaning chemicals from the school environment. Of the various healthy-schools networks forming around the country, this is the first that we are aware of that secured the active and early cooperation of school custodians—the parties most directly responsible for managing school environmental quality. Although this coalition could have been launched without custodians' support, their involvement was critical in the successful transition to safer cleaning products, and their participation can help advance the coalition's long-term agenda. In this chapter, we also review more recent projects that have employed bridge builders to organize non-unionized or self-employed workers to protect safety and health.

The bridge builders also benefit from state policies in Massachusetts that support the institutional adoption of toxics use reduction policies and makes incentives available to groups working to implement such changes. Massachusetts is not alone in this regard, however, and many other states and municipalities around the country have instituted policies that support precautionary policies such as alternatives assessment, toxics use reduction, and environmentally preferable purchasing programs [7]. Examining the Green Cleaners Project in close detail shows how organizers who are working in a specific community can leverage legislative policies and programs to extend precautionary policies and the use of environmentally friendly products to new settings.

BACKGROUND

In 1996, parents, teachers, and community activists raised a sustained protest over air quality problems in a Boston public elementary school. In response, the Boston City Council ordered the school department and the Boston Public Health Commission to conduct semi-annual environmental assessments at all Boston public schools. These inspections were not begun until 2002. The first inspection report, released in 2004, reported that 90 percent of Boston schools had at least one major environmental problem, such as leaks, poor ventilation, dust and mold, or pest incursions [8].

These issues are of concern because mold, dust, and pest dander all contribute to asthma and allergies, and Boston schools have high rates of asthma among students and staff. Asthma is the leading cause of hospitalization among children. Nationwide, it accounts for an average of 14 million missed school days each year and results in some $9 billion in health care costs; these costs may be expected to rise, as asthma rates are increasing [9]. Moreover, asthma is thought to affect attendance and overall academic performance [10]. Asthma rates in the Northeast are higher than the national average. School health records in Massachusetts show that 9.2 percent of the children have asthma [11]. Because this health burden is borne disproportionately by low-income communities and communities of color [12], the disease is a particular organizing focus among environmental justice organizations.

Cleaning products commonly contain ammonium compounds, several of which are recognized asthma triggers [13, 14]. In a survey of health care workers in four states, including Massachusetts, cleaning products were the source of the most commonly reported occupational chemical exposures linked to asthma [15]. Cleaning products are known to affect indoor air quality, also a recognized factor in exacerbation of asthma [16]. An unhealthy indoor environment in schools reduces the ability of staff to perform and of students to learn, making the reduction of asthma in Boston's public schools a priority for many stakeholders with complex and often contradictory interests.

Many of the environmental problems documented in Boston's schools, including mold, ventilation problems, and dust, are related to the age of the buildings, the choice of building materials, and school maintenance. These problems are difficult and expensive to fix. The task force therefore attempted to prioritize the issues and identify some that could be remedied cheaply and quickly. One measure was the replacement of conventional cleaning products with so-called green cleaners. The citywide task force also pressed for a policy change to require all of Boston's public schools to adopt integrated pest management, a strategy that relies primarily on nontoxic means, such as physical and mechanical barriers, to reduce insect and rodent incursions, thereby reducing the need for toxic pesticides. The school health advocates thus began with a focus on "low-hanging fruit," that is, problems that would be easy to identify, easy to reach agreement on, and easy to solve.

State-Level Efforts to Foster Precautionary Policies

Massachusetts has long been a leader in encouraging toxics reduction through statewide regulatory initiatives. The state Toxics Use Reduction Institute (TURI), established in 1989, has worked with state industries to find cost-effective and less toxic replacements for hazardous substances [17]. In 1996, TURI established the Toxics Use Reduction Networking grantmaking program (TURN) to help community organizations and municipalities develop toxics reduction programs [18]. The following year, Massachusetts passed a rule requiring all state executive departments to follow an environmentally preferable products (EPP) program designed to eliminate potential environmental and health hazards in state office buildings [19]. Policy research has documented the passage of more than 1,000 similar kinds of precautionary policies enacted in states and municipalities since 1990 [7].

A precaution-oriented philosophy has also been embraced by the Alliance for a Healthy Tomorrow. Founded in 2001, the Alliance was the first coalition in the United States to promote the precautionary principle [17], which has four central tenets: taking preventive action (even in the face of uncertainty about the scope and extent of adverse events associated with exposures); shifting the burden of proof to the proponents of an activity; widening the range of alternatives assessed; and increasing public participation in decision-making [20]. In its campaign in Boston schools, the Green Cleaners Project team has drawn on state-level efforts to foster precautionary policies (e.g., through TURI) and on a small but significant base of support in regional blue-green organizing and advocacy.

Recognizing that toxic substances to which workers are exposed in the workplace often also affect neighboring communities and the environment, the Alliance is part of a growing type of blue-green coalition focusing on protecting human health both in the workplace and the environment [6]. Previous attempts to bridge the divide between labor and environmental organizations on issues such as global warming or energy policy have typically failed to find common ground and ended in dissolution of the coalitions [2]. By focusing on health as a link between blues and greens, however, coalitions like the Alliance are forming long-lasting relationships and including a more diverse representation of environmental organizations, among them environmental health and environmental justice organizations. In their collaboration with the custodians' union in the Green Cleaners Project, Alliance members MassCOSH and BUAC have sought to establish a similar type of solidarity with workers directly affected by cleaning-chemical policies.

The Alliance has taken up the work initiated by the Green Cleaners Project team to lobby for the passage of legislation requiring use of safer products when they are available and cost-effective. The Safer Cleaning Products Bill, introduced into the Massachusetts legislature in December 2004, was designed to reduce asthma and other health threats from toxic chemicals in cleaning products by requiring that greener alternatives be used in schools, hospitals and other health care facilities, day care centers, public buildings, and public housing. The Green Cleaners Project may be seen as a test case for broader adoption of safer cleaning products, because if it is feasible for a bureaucracy as large as the Boston school system to amend purchasing strategies to adopt safer cleaning products, then it should also be possible for other large organizations to "green" their operations.

School and Health Advocacy in Boston

The Green Cleaners Project team is a special subcommittee of a citywide task force dedicated to remediating the school environmental problems identified in the 2002 environmental assessment inspections. This task force, known as the Healthy Boston Schools Project, initially comprised members of BUAC, MassCOSH, the Boston Public Health Commission, and the Boston Public School Department of Facilities Management. In the fall of 2004, BUAC was awarded a grant from TURI to review cleaning-chemical policy in Boston schools. In consultation with a MassCOSH program director, the BUAC director decided to use the city-wide task force as the base committee for this review, with the addition of representatives from the Boston school custodians' union and the school department's purchasing department. The Green Cleaners Project team thus represented various constituencies, each with a different perspective on and different responsibilities for school environmental quality. Its internal cohesion thus depended largely on bridge builders, individuals who play multiple social roles that often cross movement boundaries [21, 22].

Previous scholarship on blue-green alliances in the United States has highlighted the capacity of committee on occupational safety and health (COSH) leaders to function as bridge builders [2]. COSHes were established in the early 1970s, at a time when many unions needed to shift their focus from health and safety concerns to protecting wages and job security [23]. They readily maneuver among organizations such as unions, management, and academia and thus encourage cooperation among entities that might not otherwise collaborate [4]. MassCOSH, like other COSH groups nationwide, advocates for health and safety protection and social justice for workers [23]. In this capacity, it often works closely with union leaders, but it also engages directly with workers, community groups, and health, safety, and environmental advocates. It also represents nonunionized workers and thus functions as a surrogate union, at least with respect to workplace health and safety [4].

Founded in 1997, BUAC has sought to "promote collaboration between organizations and residents concerned about the various factors that affect asthma, such as the environment, quality of health care, access to health care, and education" [24]. BUAC's school subcommittee, comprising parents, teachers, and school employees, developed a healthy-schools platform that identifies conditions that may exacerbate asthma, such as building maintenance. Whereas most interventions in childhood asthma focus on individual treatment and management, BUAC addresses environmental causes and triggers. Like the various projects run by MassCOSH, BUAC's approach encourages cooperation among multiple stakeholders, involving school administrators, teachers, principals, custodians, and staff. This coalition may appear to not include any conventional environmental organizations, but the emergence of groups like BUAC is itself a sign of the changing face of the environmental movement. BUAC has an explicitly environmental agenda and coordinates many activities with environmental health and environmental justice groups in the area. Indeed, this "new conventionality" of environmental organizations is partly what makes blue-green coalitions possible.

Custodians in Boston public schools are organized through Local 1952 of the International Union of Painters and Allied Trades (District Council 35), representing approximately 400 full- and part-time custodians. Although the union president describes his current working relationship with the school department as cooperative and communicative, relations between the school department and the union have been difficult.

Lacking the organizational resources necessary to support a full-time health and safety committee, the custodial union worked with MassCOSH to address occupational health and safety concerns. In the early 1990s, the school department laid off approximately 50 custodians and in 1996 forced a "best and final" contract on the union that granted the school department the right to contract out custodial labor. In 2001, the school department proposed cutting more positions, leaving some small schools without a custodian on the day shift. During this round of negotiations, BUAC and MassCOSH became concerned about the effect that custodial staffing reductions would have on school environmental quality (especially with respect to waste management and integrated pest management) and collaborated with the custodial union president in an effort to preserve these jobs.

This attempt to forge a new relationship between BUAC and the custodial union, with MassCOSH continuing to provide assistance, paved the way for the subsequent collaboration on cleaning product substitution. BUAC and MassCOSH's joint organizational resources and experience in previous interactions with state environmental policies and city-level politics made them appealing as potential coalition partners to the custodians. By identifying the protection of custodial jobs as part of a larger mission to improve school environmental quality, activists at BUAC and MassCOSH also placed the issue of school environmental health in a broader context.

Framing School Health with the Logic of Precaution

This case study of multi-organizational advocacy for product substitution provides a window into how organizations negotiate a precautionary approach toward hazardous substances. Massachusetts provides institutional support for organizations to embrace toxics reduction, and there is popular support for further legislative initiatives. Nevertheless, persuading individual organizations to shift to healthier cleaning products requires stakeholders to reach a common understanding of potentially risky exposures and agree on acceptable solutions. Although the coalition partners certainly benefited from favorable political opportunities and were able to mobilize diverse resources in organizing their campaign, they also used specific discursive and rhetorical tools to align their stakeholders' concerns. The Green Cleaners Project developed a two-stage process, first demonstrating the gravity of a specific health problem and then linking its mitigation to an overall strategy of precaution. In doing so, they employed various strategies to show how the precautionary principle supported the needs and interests of different stakeholders.

Framing is a process by which social movement actors construct and maintain a common identity or arrive at an agreed-upon set of meanings that give purpose and direction to the existence and actions of a social movement organization [25, 26]. Collective-action frames are produced by social actors at various levels, from individuals to organizations to coalitions [27]. When stakeholders from multiple social movement organizations collaborate on a social problem, inter-organizational frame alignment is necessary to negotiate differences in the construction of meaning both within and between movements [26]. Whereas individual social movement organizations use frame alignment to merge the concerns of individuals into an organizational frame, coalitions use frame alignment to merge the concerns of organizations into a coalition frame.

The literature on social movements and collective action contains few case studies on the actual process of frame construction; it tends to treat frames as static elements used by social movement actors to accomplish their goals. In constructing coalition frames, aligning diverse identities and goals is particularly challenging. The differences in identity and purpose between labor unions and environmental organizations typically drive apart the interests of the groups and may explain why some blue-green coalitions have been difficult to sustain [2]. The Alliance has used the strategy of frame bridging (in which ideologically congruent yet structurally divergent frames are linked) to link environmental and occupational health. The larger coalition is thus able to draw on organizational and political support from both movements in a fundamentally new fashion. Because many of the participants in the Green Cleaners Project team were also members of the Alliance, this was a familiar strategy to them.

Frame bridging requires movement actors to agree on a common goal [26]; this agreement in turn requires specific and explicit rhetorical work to articulate a movement's goals and strategies. The Green Cleaners Project team's use of framing has both strategic and discursive properties. Strategically, frame bridging connects the interests of environmental actors and the custodial union with a specific purpose: implementing a pilot project to substitute cleaning products. It also has important movement-building implications, fostering ties across movement boundaries. In this way, the Green Cleaners Project is an example of how a social movement organization can have specific strategic goals that are reflected in a larger discursive project.

In a coalition of diverse partners, framing must also attend to the potential disconnect between individual organizations' strategic goals and those of the coalition. Furthermore, the strategic and discursive elements of a collective-action frame are not always perfectly aligned. In the Green Cleaners Project, tension arose between partners over the best methods of reaching the strategic goal of reducing asthma. Some stakeholders expressed skepticism about broadening the dialogue to include the logic of precaution. In particular, they disagreed about the extent to which the project members should invoke health problems as a rationale for endorsing a change in cleaning products, with some school administrators expecting proof of health benefits to justify a change, and the union president being reluctant to endorse actions implying that his members might face health consequences from past exposures.

While frame bridging created an opportunity to bring together specific stakeholders to facilitate a particular initiative, BUAC and MassCOSH also hoped to foster a larger project to address thornier problems of school environmental quality (e.g., mold and pest infestations). They knew that longer-term success would require building relationships between diverse actors and helping the partners appreciate that school environmental quality could be incrementally improved through short-term projects like replacing toxic cleaning products in schools with safer alternatives.

METHODS AND PROGRAM EVALUATION

The Green Cleaners Project team began by assessing products used for general cleaning, floor care, and graffiti removal. Products were screened for potential health and environmental effects. Nine of the 17 products had potential carcinogenic, teratogenic, or corrosive effects and were identified as candidates for replacement. Based on this information, the project team developed a pilot plan for the replacement of these products with "greener" alternatives.

Many of the chemical companies that produce cleaning chemicals and janitorial supplies now provide greener formulations of their regular product lines. The school department purchasing agent contacted the two companies from which Boston schools regularly purchase and ordered the greener version of all cleaning products currently used in Boston schools. A team from the facilities management department then visited the four pilot schools, removed all of the conventional formulations of the cleaning chemicals, and replaced them with the new ones. In the summer of 2004, custodians working in these schools received training in the proper use of these chemicals. Although the corporate representatives of the top cleaning-product companies typically offer training sessions to assist in the adoption of the new products, several custodians felt these corporate-sponsored training sessions to be brief and of only limited relevance in addressing the cleaning issues they faced in school environments.

With no mechanism for feedback between the custodians and product manufacturers, custodians sometimes modified the application of the green products to obtain better results and meet the demand for cleanliness. This practice may, however, compromise the safety and environmental benefits of the products or compromise product performance, if, for example, it involves applying products in heavier concentrations than the manufacturer recommends. The Green Cleaners Project team monitored the pilot program to gauge product efficacy and to make further recommendations concerning the use of green cleaning products. This evaluation included a paper-and-pencil survey of custodians in the pilot schools.

The Green Cleaners Project team also asked the Contested Illnesses Research Group (CIRG) to conduct a qualitative evaluation. Our team was happy to undertake this project, because we had a grant from the National Science Foundation to study coalition formation between labor unions and environmental organizations. Acting as consultants to the Green Cleaners Project team, we performed the qualitative evaluation and then produced a report for the team summarizing our findings. This practice is in keeping with our commitment to community-engaged advocacy and consultancy and our obligation to report findings to research participants. Twelve semi-structured interviews, ranging from 45 to 60 minutes in length, were conducted between November 2004 and February 2005 with members of the pilot team and with custodians and principals at the pilot schools. Questions covered the origins of the project, the rationale for the pilot project, expectations for evaluating the program's overall effectiveness, custodial satisfaction, and the cooperative dynamics and challenges that coalition members had experienced.

Interviews were coded and analyzed for the major themes of this project. Coding began with a pre-established set of codes, drawing on themes found in a review of the literature on school environmental health and blue-green coalitions. The code list expanded to include themes and issues that arose during the interviews, such as framing of the health message and brokering of negotiations. Transcripts were analyzed by the first and second authors of this chapter; unreferenced quotations are drawn directly from interview transcripts. We submitted a short report of our findings to the Green Cleaners Product team, which was used in the overall evaluation of the pilot program.

The Green Cleaners Pilot Project is the first application of the blue-green model in an institution like education, where diverse stakeholders might be brought together to address concerns about protecting human health and the environment. However, because this type of collaboration between custodians, environmentalists, and children's health activists is rare, we are limited in the extent to which we can generalize from this study until further examples can be identified and analyzed.

RESULTS

The Green Cleaners Project team succeeded in persuading school administrators to shift to green cleaners for two main reasons. First, the team successfully bridged the typically oppositional concerns of multiple and diverse stakeholders, effectively neutralizing the objections or securing the support of those that might have made such a project infeasible. By enlisting the custodial union as participants in the pilot project, the Green Cleaners Project team was able to convince the union that the initiative to switch cleaning products would not threaten jobs, that it would strengthen the union's calls for better worker training in general, and that it would allow custodians to participate in decisions about their work environment. The coalition thus strategically circumvented potential opposition to environmental initiatives on the grounds that they would threaten jobs. Second, the team developed and maintained a strategic frame for this project that unified the health concerns of school staff, environmental health activists, and the custodians' union under the umbrella of the precautionary principle. The project ultimately addressed both the community's and activists' concerns about health and school environmental quality and the workers' concerns about workplace safety and training. These two strategies helped to secure the participation of the major stakeholders in this coalition and have laid the groundwork for future collaborations among this team on other issues in school environmental health.

Enlisting Custodians in Protecting School Environmental Health

MassCOSH's organizational role was vital to the Green Cleaners Project, and its program director was an essential bridge builder. She is a founding member of BUAC and also heads the BUAC school health committee and chairs MassCOSH's Healthy Schools Network. Through her involvement with the MassCOSH and BUAC school health committees, she had extensive knowledge of the environmental issues in Boston schools and strong personal contacts with decision-makers in the school administration as well as with the leaders of the teachers' and custodial unions. Her previous interaction with the custodial union helped establish the communication necessary for successful bridge building. Her involvement in the Alliance allowed her to apply the logic and discourse of precaution as a central element in the construction of the coalition frame, and her leadership in the Alliance and in the statewide Healthy Schools Network enabled her to link a local campaign for school environmental health to wider initiatives. Thus from the outset, the Green Cleaners Project had advantages in city and statewide politics, both in terms of access to political officials and in familiarity with the advocacy efforts of one of the state's most visible environmental coalitions.

The MassCOSH program director was well aware that the custodial union needed an advocate to support its initiatives to improve worker health and employee training. For the custodial union, job security and wages are paramount; it lacks the bargaining power to make health issues a priority. The custodial union president had first met the MassCOSH and BUAC organizers at city-wide hearings when the school administration proposed eliminating custodial jobs. The president expressed his members' longstanding frustrations in their jobs. He noted, for example, that his members bristle at the use of the term *dirty* to describe the schools: "When people walk into a building and they see like, the plaster falling down and stuff, they perceive that as being dirty, so they blame the custodian, so we should be involved to really explain what the problem is, instead. Because people just see certain things and say, 'Oh, that's dirt.' But what's causing that?" The custodial union has struggled to gain recognition of the structural problems that contribute to school environmental quality, such as staffing, funding, and capital plans for building maintenance.

The MassCOSH project leader understood and acknowledged this position: "There has been a lot of shuffling around and staff reduction, too. . . . Some of the small schools didn't have custodians for some of the key hours of the school day, so if a kid threw up, the teacher either threw something, like that kitty litter stuff, on it, and they would call a floater custodian to come and clean it, or it would wait until they had their part-time person after school come and clean it. And we just felt like that was a public health problem." The union president appreciated MassCOSH's support at these hearings to help him hold the line against further job cuts. He was willing to cooperate on the Green Cleaners Project because he perceived MassCOSH as an important external advocate that could augment the union's efforts to protect jobs and to advocate for members' health and increased worker training.

The school department's decision to shift to green cleaners included a renewed commitment to worker training and an agreement to form a standing committee for the periodic review of cleaning-chemical use in schools, which would include a representative from the custodial union. These two provisions were significant victories for the Green Cleaners Project team. School administrators interviewed for this project reported that the chemical manufacturers all offer a range of products that change frequently. They had changed product formulations frequently in the past, but before this project began, they had not sought input or feedback on these decisions from the custodians. Although janitorial work has historically been considered semi-skilled labor, over the past several decades, as the global economy has tightened, labor markets and more and more organizations have contracted out janitorial services, the work has been transformed into low-skilled, low-wage "dirty" work. The reliance on part-time and unskilled laborers has often driven contract cleaning companies to select cleaners based on their potency and efficacy, in an effort to curb costs by avoiding the need for worker training [28].

The evaluation of green cleaning products in the Green Cleaners pilot project included several types of qualitative assessment of product performance and the custodians' job satisfaction. Several custodians identified practical barriers to using green products, notably lack of equipment or insufficient training. Custodians expressed some dissatisfaction with several of the new products, but on investigation it was discovered that the custodians were using the products inappropriately (e.g., at full strength rather than diluted). This finding highlights the importance of active participation by the labor union in decisions about product substitution, and the need for training in product use.

Previous studies of janitorial work have demonstrated that management often pursues a combination of strategies (including job speed-up or work restructuring) to de-skill custodial work and to thereby justify harsh labor practices and low pay. Pressure by workers and labor activists for training for custodial workforces is therefore not motivated purely by concerns about occupational health but may also be seen as an effort to defend custodial work as semi-skilled labor and thus to restore the dignity of the workers and their right to a living wage [28, 29]. MassCOSH and the union made worker training and worker input into chemical performance and selection an integral part of the campaign. The presence of MassCOSH as a strong and well-established labor advocate on the project team brought a strong pro-labor voice to the table.

Throughout the pilot evaluation, participation in decision-making was a significant issue. School administrators preferred to see the review of cleaning products as a case of top-down decision-making, whereas other partners, like MassCOSH and the custodial union, pressed for greater involvement by those using the products. In the words of one school department official, the discussion of shifting to green cleaning products prompted further discussion about school cleaning chemical policies "among ourselves [administrators], which is probably where it belongs anyway." The custodian association president rather pessimistically stated that regardless of the decisions made about the Green Cleaners Project, custodians would have to use whatever products the school department provided. This view was echoed by the custodians in the pilot schools, who universally indicated that they had no input into product selection. Without advocacy by the BUAC and MassCOSH partners, it is unlikely that any call for a review of cleaning products would have arisen from the workforce or been heeded by management. In some respects, then, the greatest success of the Green Cleaners Project team may have been in obtaining employee input into decisions.

Bridge building operates largely through communication, and in particular by communication across the labor-environmental divide. MassCOSH was able to persuade the custodial union of the benefits of adopting a precautionary framework for school environmental health not so much on the strength of claims about alternatives assessment and product substitution as because of the way it democratizes decision-making about toxic exposures. This element of the campaign aligned with the strategies of the custodial union in bargaining for training and participation in decision-making.

Maintaining a Comprehensive Coalition Frame

Framing is essential if a social movement organization is to communicate its goals effectively, both among its membership and to political decision-makers. For cross-movement coalitions such as labor-environmental partnerships, identifying common ground is especially important. Collaborations that link diverse organizations often take modest initial steps whose feasibility and success demonstrate the potential of a long-term collaboration. The Green Cleaners Project team leaders articulated this strategy consciously. By focusing initially on a high-profile school health problem such as asthma, and targeting the substitution of greener cleaning chemicals as a simple solution agreeable to all stakeholders, the team sought to create a solid base for a coalition that would integrate the concerns of school administrators and teachers, custodians, students, and parents; establish the merit of a precautionary approach to school health issues; and lay a foundation for future campaigns to improve school environmental quality.

The project leaders began their framing efforts by emphasizing the significance of asthma as a school health issue, suggesting that traditional cleaning products presented hazards to both employees and students. However, the lack of data that link product substitution and improved health created some difficulties in getting all parties to agree on a common set of evaluation criteria. Thus project participants faced a challenge in establishing clear evaluation standards and setting goals that would show how switching cleaning products would clearly advance the overall goal of improving school environmental health. Several members of the project team, for example, said that they thought the ultimate decision about whether the school system should shift to green cleaners should be made on the basis of whether asthma was actually reduced among students in the pilot schools: if such data were not available, then cost-effectiveness should carry the day.

The project leaders had hoped to sidestep controversies over the lack of data by including in the framing of the project an orientation toward a broader prevention-based, or precautionary, approach. Although they believed they established the shift to a precautionary stance as the ultimate goal of the project, several members of the committee (especially the school administrators) insisted that because the project had begun with a specific discussion of asthma as a school health issue, they should expect quantifiable evidence that the program was improving asthma outcomes. This problem persisted despite repeated cautions from other members of the team that the project did not include monitoring for a decline in asthma incidence. These misconceptions suggested that the lack of agreement on evaluation metrics persisted and that at least some members of the team were in disagreement about the adequacy of a precautionary approach as a discursive frame to address this potential health issue.

Members of the project team also disagreed about whether the potential health risks associated with cleaning products should be the chief articulation of the coalition's central issue. Although the two women leading the project (representing BUAC and MassCOSH) wanted to maintain a focus on health, the custodial union president expressed concern: "If it's an issue, I have no problem making it a major issue, but if it's not an issue, I don't really want to scare people about it. But I think if we just explain that in the long term, these chemicals will be healthier, easy to use, you don't have to worry if you spill it on you. I mean, some of the chemicals, like the strippers, if you put it on your hand and didn't wash it off, you got a burn. Stuff like that. If you use different chemicals, you might not have to worry about that."

This ambivalence represents a legitimate concern on the part of workers: some of the union members had worked with these potentially hazardous products for a long time, and the union head did not want to raise concerns about past exposures. In the end, however, he supported the product-substitution effort because of the broader discursive framing of the campaign, which included the democratizing principles of participation in decision-making. Moreover, he reported a shift in his attitude over the course of the project. After the school department announced that they would shift to green cleaning products, he reported his pleasure at this outcome and his appreciation for the assistance the union had received from MassCOSH and BUAC. On seeing how powerful health messages and a precautionary approach can be in articulating problems, he described himself as being more open to collaboration with other healthy-school advocates.

The union president's initial ambivalence about conveying a strong health message may have been communicated to the custodians, however, when they were trained in using the new products. When the custodians in the pilot schools were asked by researchers why they thought the school system had shifted to these newer cleaning products, two recalled having been told that the products were safer or healthier for themselves and the students; the other two replied that they thought the shift had been made to save storage space or because the new products were cheaper. The two janitors who were aware of the health-based rationale for product substitution also had more favorable impressions of the new products. One of these custodians has asthma and appreciated the new products because, unlike the old products, they did not induce wheezing. In contrast, the two custodians who believed the shift had been made for other reasons were more critical of the products' performance and indicated that decisions on shifting to green cleaners should be made on the basis of cost. Custodians' lack of awareness about the importance of health in making the shift to green cleaners may have influenced their assessment of the new products, as their application often differs significantly from that of traditional products and requires more physical labor.

The connection between the strategic aims of the cleaning-products substitution project and the discursive project drawing attention to school environmental health problems was perceived best by individuals who were themselves suffering from health problems. Custodians who suffered from asthma were more likely to connect the project with the larger goal of improving health, whereas custodians who perceived themselves to be in good health and unaffected by the traditional cleaning products viewed the pilot project as a simple administrative shift in the materials they were instructed to use. Thus, if personal experience mediates the acceptance of a coalition frame, organizers should decide which parts of the frame or message need to be made explicit.

The challenge of constructing a coalition collective-action frame for this project demonstrates that even when all parties have a stake in creating and maintaining a healthy school environment, they may approach the problem from different angles, with different understandings of the scope of the problem and different goals for remediation. More opportunities for engaged and participatory discussions of environmental quality early in the process could have helped in clarifying the goals and positions of all stakeholders, in enumerating and prioritizing environmental problems, and in developing a plan that satisfied the interests of all stakeholders. Candid and frequent discussion of how short-term projects relate to overall long-term strategies is also important.

DISCUSSION

The Green Cleaners Project's alliance of environmental health and labor activists, workers, and school administrators is a model other school districts can follow to foster a healthy environment for students and staff. By building a coalition among multiple stakeholders, all of whom have a material interest in managing school environmental quality, the project leaders were able to mitigate or neutralize ideological divisions that have traditionally scuttled cooperative efforts between labor and environmental movement organizations.

The participation of such a varied group of participants demanded the construction of a robust coalition frame. The precautionary principle made a good basis for this frame because team members could match its tenets to the environmental health activists' interest in product substitution as well as to the union's objectives of improving worker training and expanding workers' participation in decision-making. The Green Cleaners Project provides a model for building new forms of labor-environmental coalitions, with bridge-building organizations such as MassCOSH occupying a critical role in mediation.

The project leaders were careful in framing the issues in this project: first, they selected a high-profile health issue, student asthma, to stimulate a wider debate about school environmental quality; and second, they invoked a philosophy of precaution as a means of mitigating the problem. This strategy allowed them to gain the attention of school officials by invoking a well-documented student health problem, and then to fold in a latent concern about the effect of cleaning products on workers' health. It is unlikely that the custodial union would have been effective in challenging decisions about the selection of cleaning products because of its relatively weak bargaining position.

The second strategy, framing the issue from a precautionary standpoint, allowed the team leaders to sidestep problems of demonstrating improved health outcomes in the absence of quantifiable data. However, a tension emerged between the more strategically oriented frame of reducing asthma and the broader discursive framing in favor of precaution-based environmental health policies. Nevertheless, setting the initial objective of product substitution allowed project leaders to link this campaign to larger campaigns at the state and national levels that invoke precaution as a rationale for improving and protecting school environmental quality.

Constructing a coalition frame that is broad enough to address and support the individual and common needs of a variety of organizations is a delicate process, and the experience of this team points to some clear deficiencies in theories of frame development and maintenance. The project leaders relied on the logic of the precautionary principle because they believed its tenets could unify the disparate needs of the coalition partners. In practice, this meant that they relied on some elements of precaution in conversations with some coalition members more than in discussions with others, especially in the early, crucial stages of coalition formation. The fact that not all coalition members readily embraced all elements of the principle (the union president was initially hesitant, and school administrators were resistant throughout the process) might suggest that the attempt to bridge the frames of the coalition partners was not wholly successful, even though the coalition did achieve its goal of product substitution. Theories of frame bridging and alignment need to be expanded to help us understand how and when coalition partners activate or rely on particular strategic or discursive elements of the frame in bringing coalition partners together. More theoretical work is also needed to help us understand how and when a coalition can persist and succeed when not all members have embraced all the elements of a complex frame, and how and when it might fail entirely. Though here we have stressed the importance of framing over more structural elements, building solidarity between labor and environmental organizations involves finding both a common ideological frame and the structural means to allow the groups to work together. By building ties through the promotion of the precautionary principle, the coalition leaders tied the concept of prevention to the more concrete goals of democratic decision-making and increased worker and community control over working conditions.

As existing school infrastructure continues to deteriorate and funding remains inadequate, school environmental quality will become a greater problem for schools nationwide. The model of collaboration between diverse stakeholders adopted in Boston can serve as an example for other health and safety activists. Concerns are growing about toxic exposures for service-sector workers [28]. From the perspective of labor unions and worker organizations seeking new issues to emphasize in organizing campaigns [30], health and safety and the environment are becoming central issues [2, 5]. Furthermore, by arguing that workers should have a voice in decisions about the selection of products they use on a daily basis, campaigns such as the Green Cleaners Project are also advocating for worker empowerment and a larger role in decision-making.

This program also highlights challenges and pitfalls that may beset blue-green or school–environmental health coalitions. Although the team had some success in integrating the concerns of school administrators, custodians, and environmental health groups, some stakeholders were absent from the discussions: other school employees, such as kitchen and cafeteria workers; teachers; and parents. All these groups are affected by and can influence the implementation and effectiveness of new policies. BUAC has been particularly successful in enlisting parent advocates, for example by training them to testify in support of various pieces of legislation. Parents should be briefed on the green cleaners program so that they can advocate for healthier school policies locally and statewide. Although including additional stakeholders in the process could complicate the decision-making process, it could also strengthen awareness of school environmental problems and enhance the community's commitment to school environmental health.

MassCOSH as a Bridge Builder

MassCOSH's involvement in the Green Cleaners Project was critical in enlisting the support and participation of all stakeholders throughout the process and led to the achievement of three practical objectives. First, the project team leaders pressed the school department for a commitment to train custodians in the proper use of new products. The custodial union had long demanded improved training for its workers but had needed to subordinate these demands to their efforts to protect jobs and wages. Second, the formalization of this Green Cleaners Project through the citywide school health task force provided a mechanism for detection of health problems in the schools in the future and a forum in which these problems could be discussed and solutions could be entertained. Finally, the cooperation of the custodial union with labor advocates and environmental health activists laid the groundwork for future collaborations in which custodians can document the persistence or emergence of problems that threaten school environmental quality. Although there are other healthy-schools programs around the country, the Massachusetts project is among the few that includes custodial unions as core partners.

Coalition Building among Non-unionized Workers

Since the success of the Green Cleaners Project, MassCOSH has continued its work in lobbying for toxics-use reduction and expanded its organizing role by advocating for legislative and administrative policies and practices that protect non-unionized workers. This work has included policy advocacy to craft new regulations to protect workers, and supporting self-employed workers in environmentally preferable purchasing initiatives.

In 2005, two house fires in the Boston area occurred while hardwood floors were being sanded and refinished. Both fires resulted in the deaths of three Vietnamese workers who were working with highly toxic and flammable lacquer-based floor-finishing products. Over the past decade, more than two dozen similar fires have occurred in the Boston area, leading to more than a million dollars' worth of property damage. In response to these episodes, MassCOSH convened a working group that brought together chemical suppliers, distributors, and representatives from the community of independent contractors who work with these chemicals. This working group received consulting support from TURI, which evaluated the lacquer-based chemicals used in floor sanding and refinishing processes and identified safer, readily available water-based alternatives. They issued a white paper summarizing their findings, conducted education and outreach among the contractors who apply these chemicals (many of whom are Vietnamese or Cape Verdean), and convened a task force that would advise on the development of legislation to regulate the chemicals in use in this industry [31].

The task force meetings were important in bringing together representatives from the major chemical suppliers and distributors in a forum where they could all agree on the dangers involved in the continued use of the lacquer-based chemicals. In the absence of legislation banning the products, a joint pledge to withdraw them from the market simultaneously (so that no supplier or distributor would retain a competitive advantage) was an important step in protecting the health of the contractors. Perhaps predictably, some contractors objected, because lacquer-based chemicals allow them to work more quickly. But through the task force, suppliers, distributors, and contractors could agree on the hazards posed by these products and the process of withdrawing them, both to protect worker health and safety and to create a level playing field for the other stakeholders [31].

As in the Green Cleaners Project, MassCOSH played an important role as a bridge builder. The task was more complex in this instance, partly because of the decentralized and non-unionized workforce but also because the involvement of the business community was different. Many more small decision-makers needed to be persuaded to change their purchasing practices, as opposed to a central purchasing office in a school bureaucracy. This project also marked the first time that MassCOSH worked directly with business owners (the chemical suppliers and distributors), and the project leader was initially anxious that those parties might attempt to stonewall efforts at product substitution. In the end, however, this concern was unfounded, perhaps because of the highly public and tragic incidents that triggered the task force's formation.

MassCOSH's strategy of bringing together diverse stakeholders—academic health and safety experts from TURI, the chemical suppliers, the distributors, and the independent contractors—enhanced the task force's credibility and led to their success in securing informal agreements to protect workers that would later be codified formally. Task force members reached out to influential policy-makers to educate them about this problem, and enacted state-level policy changes. In June 2010, the Massachusetts State Fire Marshal's office revised parts of the fire code to incorporate this knowledge about the dangers of flammable floor finishing products in their permitting and safety requirements [32]. The Massachusetts legislature passed a bill in 2010 prohibiting the sale and use of the most hazardous chemicals used in floor finishing and to ensure worker training in the proper application of the safer formulations of these chemicals [33].

In similar fashion, MassCOSH has sought to promote toxics use reduction by supporting small business owners who wish to adopt safer chemical practices. MassCOSH has long been a partner in two university-community partnerships that focus on immigrant health: Project COBWEB (Collaboration for a Better Work Environment for Brazilians, based out of the University of Massachusetts–Lowell) and Assessing and Controlling Occupational Health Risks to Immigrants in Somerville (led by researchers from Tufts University). Both academic teams receive funding from the National Institute of Environmental Health Sciences [34]. Both projects take a participatory action research approach to empowering communities to identify occupational and environmental hazards and organize to remediate them. Through outreach with Brazilian housecleaners in the Boston area, community organizers identified exposure to household cleaning chemicals as a potential threat to worker safety and health. Housecleaning is a common occupation for Brazilian women in the Boston area, but the isolated nature of the work renders women vulnerable to a range of health and safety hazards [35]. Organizers helped a group of house cleaners band together to form a worker's cooperative that purchases green cleaning chemicals in bulk for its members. The cooperative leaders reported a reduction in symptoms associated with the use of conventional cleaning products and an enhanced sense of mutual support for other workers [35]. Through similar projects, MassCOSH has helped train cosmetologists in exposure-reduction practices to protect them and their clients from noxious fumes in beauty salons.

CONCLUSION

What began as a pilot project to substitute cleaning products in Boston's schools has raised some provocative questions about coalition formation. The bridge-building and framing strategies that the organizers employed here may be useful for blue-green coalitions and coalitions working to address occupational health, in schools but also in other settings. In the examples shown here, the precautionary principle has served as a frame flexible enough to meet the needs of environmental health activists, while also fulfilling labor's desire for participatory decision-making in matters of occupational health and social justice. Supporting an institutionalized home for the precautionary principle in state policy has been an ongoing challenge in the wake of the recent economic downturn, however. In 2009, the legislature proposed drastic cuts to TURI's budget, which would have compromised its ability to support businesses and communities in alternatives assessment. The continued work of the Alliance and MassCOSH to keep chemicals policy on the agenda of state bureaus and the Massachusetts legislature could quite possibly have helped in resisting these efforts to cut TURI's budget. This research also suggests that organizations may fulfill a bridge-building role in the formation of coalitions, at least in ones that include labor activists and labor unionists. More work is needed to determine how, whether, and when coalitions decide to adopt the logic of precaution; how it affects the composition of the coalition; and how it contributes to a coalition's success.

Perhaps most importantly, research like this highlights the need for multidisciplinary studies of public health problems. Public health professionals are paying greater attention to how indoor environments affect health; this research has identified threats from indoor air quality, unsafe equipment, and lifting hazards [36, 37]. But this research should engage not only industrial hygienists who work to characterize the specific threats that exist in indoor environments, but should also integrate social scientists, community activists, and affected individuals. Understanding the perspectives of workers who are most directly impacted by hazards is critical to understanding how power dynamics in the workplace continue to subject workers to hazards and threaten health and safety [38].

ACKNOWLEDGMENTS

This work was supported in part by the National Science Foundation Program in Social Dimensions of Engineering, Science, and Technology (Grant # SES-0350691) and the National Science Foundation Program in Sociology (Grant # SES-0401869). The authors thank Rebecca Gasior Altman and Heleneke Mulder for their valuable comments. We also thank the Boston Urban Asthma Coalition, the Boston School Department, the International Union of Painters and Allied Trades District Council Number 35, and the Massachusetts Committee on Occupational Safety and Health for their cooperation and collaboration in this work.

This work is adapted from a version published in *Contested Illnesses: Citizens, Science, and Health Social Movements*, edited by Phil Brown, Rachel Morello-Frosch, Stephen Zavestoski, and the Contested Illnesses Research Group (Berkeley and Los Angeles, CA: University of California Press, 2011).

NOTES

1. Center for Health, Environment, and Justice, *Creating Safe Learning Zones: The ABCs of Healthy Schools*, 2002.
2. Brian Obach, *Labor and the Environmental Movement: The Quest for Common Ground.* (Cambridge, MA: MIT Press, 2004).
3. Brian Mayer, *Blue-Green Coalitions: Fighting for Safe Workplaces and Healthy Communities* (Ithaca, NY: Cornell ILR Press, 2008).
4. Robert Gottlieb, *Forcing the Spring: The Transformation of the American Environmental Movement* (revised and updated edition) (Washington, D.C.: Island Press, 2005).
5. K. A. Gould, T. Lewis, and J. T. Roberts, "Blue-Green Coalitions: Constraints and Possibilities in the Post 9-11 Political Environment," *Journal of World-Systems Research* 10(1) (2004): 91-116.
6. Brian Mayer and Phil Brown, "Constructing a Coalition Frame in a Cross-Movement Coalition: New Jersey's Labor-Environmental Alliance," Annual Conference, American Sociological Association, Philadelphia, PA, 2005.
7. Northeast Waste Management Officials' Association, Interstate Chemicals Clearinghouse, State Chemicals Policy Database, http://www.newmoa.org/prevention/ic2/projects/chempolicy/ (accessed September 21, 2012).
8. Tracy Jan, "Environmental Report Details City School Ills," *Boston Globe*, November 19, 2004.
9. American Lung Association, *Children and Asthma in America*, 2004.
10. M. J. Mendell and G. A. Heath, "Do Indoor Air Pollutants and Thermal Conditions in Schools Influence Student Performance? A Critical Review of the Literature," *Indoor Air* 15(1) (2005): 27-52.

11. R. S. Knorr et al., "Tracking Pediatric Asthma: The Massachusetts Experience Using School Health Records," *Environmental Health Perspectives* 112 (2004): 1424-1427.
12. B. Bloom et al., "Summary Health Statistics for U.S. Children: National Health Interview Survey, 2001," *Vital Health Statistics 10* (2003): 1-54.
13. J. A. Bernstein et al., "A Combined Respiratory and Cutaneous Hypersensitivity Syndrome Induced by Work Exposure to Quaternary Amines," *Journal of Allergy and Clinical Immunology* 94(2 Pt. 1) (1994): 257-259.
14. A. Purohit et al., "Quaternary Ammonium Compounds and Occupational Asthma," *International Archives of Occupational and Environmental Health* 73(6) (2000): 423-427.
15. E. Pechter et al., "Work-Related Asthma among Health Care Workers: Surveillance Data from California, Massachusetts, Michigan, and New Jersey, 1993-1997," *American Journal of Industrial Medicine* 47 (2005): 265-275.
16. D. Shendell, C. Barnett, and S. Boese, "Science-Based Recommendations to Prevent or Reduce Potential Exposure to Biological, Chemical, and Physical Agents in Schools," *Journal of School Health* 74(10) (2004): 390-396.
17. B. Mayer, P. Brown, and M. Linder, "Moving Further Upstream: From Toxics Reduction to the Precautionary Principle," *Public Health Reports* 117 (2002): 574-586.
18. Toxics Use Reduction Institute, *TURNing Partnerships into Progress in Massachusetts Communities: A Retrospective of the Toxics Use Reduction Networking (TURN) Grantmaking Program*, 2003.
19. Code of Massachusetts Regulations, Procurement of Commodities or Services, Including Human and Social Services, 801 CMR 21.00.
20. D. Kriebel et al., "The Precautionary Principle in Environmental Science," *Environmental Health Perspectives* 109 (2001): 871-876.
21. B. Robnett, "African-American Women in the Civil Rights Movement, 1954-1965: Gender, Leadership, and Micromobilization," *American Journal of Sociology* 101(6) (1981): 1661-1693.
22. Fred Rose, *Coalitions across the Class Divide: Lessons from the Labor, Peace, and Environmental Movements* (Ithaca, NY: Cornell University Press, 2000).
23. D. Berman, "Grassroots Coalitions in Health and Safety: The COSH Groups," *Labor Studies Journal* Spring (1981): 104-113.
24. Boston Urban Asthma Coalition, "The BUAC Mission," www.buac.org/about_us.html (accessed August 31, 2006).
25. Donnatella Della Porta and Mario Diani, *Social Movements: An Introduction* (Oxford: Blackwell Publishing, 1999).
26. R. Benford and D. A. Snow, "Framing Processes and Social Movements: An Overview and Assessment," *Annual Review of Sociology* 26 (2000): 611-639.
27. D. Croteau and L. Hicks, "Coalition Framing and the Challenge of a Consonant Frame Pyramid: The Case of a Collaborative Response to Homelessness," *Social Problems* 50 (2003): 251-172.
28. Robert Gottlieb, *Environmentalism Unbound: Exploring New Pathways for Change.* (Cambridge, MA: MIT Press, 2001).
29. Leslie Salzinger, "A Maid by Any Other Name: The Transformation of 'Dirty Work' by Central American Immigrants," in *Ethnography Unbound: Power and Resistance in the Modern Metropolis*, ed. M. Burawoy (Berkeley, CA: University of California Press, 1991) 139-160.

30. Dan Clawson, *The Next Upsurge: Labor and the New Social Movements* (Ithaca, NY: Cornell University Press, 2003).
31. L. Azaroff et al., "Results of a Community-University Partnership to Reduce Deadly Hazards in Hardwood Floor Finishing," *Journal of Community Health* 36 (2011): 658-668.
32. Code of Massachusetts Regulations, Board of Fire Prevention Regulations, Floor Finishing or Refinishing, 57 CMR 10.15.
33. Massachusetts General Laws, Sale, possession, or use of lacquer sealer prohibited; penalties. Chapter 94, Section 329.
34. C. E. Siqueira, "Community-Engaged Environmental Justice Research at University of Massachusetts Lowell," *American Journal of Public Health* 99(S3) (2009): S485-S487.
35. D. M. Gute et al., "The Viva Verde Women's Co-Op: Brazilian Immigrants Organizing to Promote Environmental and Social Justice," *American Journal of Public Health* 99(S3) (2009): S495-S498.
36. M. F. Flum et al., "Photovoice in the Workplace: A Participatory Method to Give Voice to Workers to Identify Health and Safety Hazards and Promote Workplace Change—A Study of University Custodians," *American Journal of Industrial Medicine* 53 (2010): 1150-1158.
37. Paula Schenck et al., "A Coordinated Program of On-Going Risk Communication, Adult and Student Health Surveys, Interim Intervention, and Engineering Oversight to Manage Indoor Air Quality Concerns at a School" Annual Meeting, American Public Health Association, November 15-19, 2003.
38. D. D. Biehler and G. L. Simon, "The Great Indoors: Research Frontiers on Indoor Environments as Active Political-Ecological Spaces," *Progress in Human Geography* 35(2) (2010): 172-192.

PART III

Advances in Policy

CHAPTER 11

Integrated Pest Management Policies in America's Schools: Is Federal Legislation Needed?

Andrea Kidd Taylor, Kyle Esdaille, and Jennifer Ames

America's schoolchildren and adults who work in schools are at risk of developing asthma and other respiratory illnesses as a result of exposure to hazardous pesticides. Integrated pest management (IPM) policies are being implemented in states and school districts across the country; however, the content and regulation of these policies vary. Standardization of such policies through a federal IPM law is the only way to ensure that children and workers in America's schools are adequately protected from exposure to hazardous pesticides used to control pests.

In school environments across the United States, pests can be major sources of indoor allergens. High-traffic areas where food is prepared, stored, and served—along with areas where trash accumulates or where water is stagnant—are perfect breeding grounds for a variety of pests, including ants, cockroaches, termites, mice, and rats. Children are particularly vulnerable to pest allergens, and they spend a large portion of their time in schools. Many studies document the hazards of childhood exposure to pests, particularly risks of respiratory illnesses such as asthma and other breathing problems [1]. In an effort to control pests and reduce pest problems in schools, and to reduce children's and workers' exposures to pests, school administrators have often resorted to traditional pest control methods consisting of harmful pesticides in these indoor environments, thereby creating additional health risks and exacerbating respiratory illnesses, particularly asthma, in children and adults [2]. According to the scientific literature, pesticides have a negative effect on the respiratory, endocrine, neurological, and immune systems of children and adults, even at low doses [3, 4].

A 2005 study published in the *Journal of the American Medical Association* (*JAMA*) found higher incident rates of acute pesticide-related illness among school employees than among children between 1998 and 2002 using data from three different national surveillance systems. Those affected included individuals who handled pesticides (custodians, gardeners, food preparation workers, and teachers) as well as those who did not handle pesticides and were exposed on school grounds. The authors note that the lack of a single national surveillance system and the inconsistency of surveillance methods at the state level probably lead to significant underreporting of pesticide poisoning in school environments [5]. In an attempt to reduce pests and children's exposure to pesticides, integrated pest management (IPM) policies are being implemented in schools, local communities, and states across the country.

The definition of IPM varies widely; however, the major principle of IPM is to use alternative methods for controlling pests and to use the least toxic pesticides only as a last resort [6]. Many school IPM policies have similar language and guidelines; however, the adoption and implementation of these policies vary widely nationwide—from school to school, school district to school district, and state to state. Given the inconsistencies in the implementation of current IPM policies, some environmental advocates have called for federal legislation to better protect children from exposure to harmful pesticides.

BACKGROUND AND IPM DEFINITIONS

As early as the 1970s, the California State Parent Teacher Association (PTA) recognized the harmful health effects of childhood exposure to pesticides and passed a resolution calling for reduced use of pesticides in schools [7]. The California PTA's efforts and resolution sparked the interests and efforts of the National Parent Association, the National Education Association, and other public interest organizations around the country to support the implementation of IPM policies and reduce pesticide use in schools. The California Healthy Schools Act, passed in 2000, requires schools to designate an IPM coordinator, notify parents in advance of pesticide use, and maintain public records of pesticide application [8]. In the state of Maryland, the school IPM legislation passed in 1997 was spearheaded by the Maryland Pesticide Network, a public interest organization [9]. In both places, IPM is defined as pest management strategies that use safer methods, including sanitation, nonchemical agents, biological agents, structural repairs, and mechanical and physical controls to prevent, monitor, and treat pest problems. Only after failure of these methods should the least toxic/harmful pesticides be used [4, 7]. The main controversy surrounding most IPM definitions is what constitutes the "least toxic" or "least harmful" pesticide or chemical and whether the use of any pesticide or chemical is necessary to control pest infestation. Across the nation, inconsistencies in the adoption and implementation of integrated pest management policies may be due to how IPM

is defined, interpreted and understood, and practiced. Integrated pest management may be defined as any method that effectively prevents, mitigates, or evaluates pest infestations without the use of toxic chemicals.

Most local and state IPM policies include three or more of the following components: 1) formal notification to parents, staff, and students prior to any pesticide application; 2) training and education for IPM personnel; 3) posting of warning signs for pesticide applications; 4) accurate recordkeeping of all pesticides used; and 5) access to material safety data sheets (MSDSs) that include the chemical identity of the pesticides used [4, 6, 10-14].

PRACTICES OF PROFESSIONAL PEST CONTROL CONTRACTORS AND SCHOOL ADMINISTRATORS

Many pest management professionals (PMPs) or contractors tend to apply more pesticides than necessary to control pests; and many feel constrained by using IPM techniques [15]. Unfortunately, very often school administrators hire and rely on PMPs to control pests in their schools. In a North Carolina State University study, a focus group and telephone survey of PMPs with school contracts in North Carolina were conducted to determine pest control practices and PMPs' understanding and use of IPM. From the focus group and survey, several constraints and barriers to PMPs' adopting and fully practicing IPM were identified [15]:

1. skepticism about the effectiveness of IPM;
2. lack of understanding by school administrators and staff that IPM programs require partnership and good communication;
3. school occupants having a low tolerance to pests and considering every pest sighting as an emergency;
4. the selection of different contractors on a "low bidder" basis and poor contract management;
5. the complexity of school structures and their accessibility for pest control;
6. liability issues related to pest control and the sensitivity of school occupants;
7. lack of motivation of PMPs to use IPM;
8. lack of clarity of the definition and objectives of IPM; and
9. lack of IPM education and training.

PMPs are usually certified professionals, and many feel that pests are only controlled by the application of pesticides [15].

Efforts are ongoing to change the thinking and practices of PMPs and pest control companies who believe that the more conventional methods of applying pesticides to control pests are the only means of addressing pest problems in the school environment. In fact, a few studies indicate that IPM practices are more effective than the conventional methods used to control pests, and that the major requirements for influencing changes in current pesticide application practices are the use of better cleaning and sanitation methods, more training and education, and better communication [1, 3]. One such study, the first of its kind to evaluate the effectiveness of conventional pest control methods and IPM in controlling cockroach infestations and cockroach allergens in schools, found that the IPM approach was more effective at reducing cockroach infestation and allergen levels than the conventional approach (routine, calendar-based pesticide applications) [1]. Many researchers have provided evidence that IPM programs are more effective than conventional pest control methods, and IPM can lead to long-term reductions in pest allergens in school environments, thereby providing a healthier school environment for teachers, administrators, staff, and students.

CURRENT IPM POLICIES AND PROBLEMS

School IPM policies vary widely nationwide. Many state school IPM policies are voluntary. In some states, the jurisdiction for pest control and IPM laws is within the states' agriculture departments; in others, within the states' health departments and/or environmental protection departments or agencies. Furthermore, variation across states' IPM policies in terms of record-keeping, enforcement and implementation has made it difficult for researchers to make meaningful comparisons across IPM policies and evaluate their relative efficacy [5].

A few state pest control policies mainly address licensing and certification of pesticide applicators [16-24]. Beyond Pesticides (formerly the National Coalition Against the Misuse of Pesticides), an independent advocacy organization, works with other environmental organizations and allies to protect public health and the environment by leading the call for transitioning to a world free of toxic pesticides. Beyond Pesticides (BP) maintains the most up-to-date and detailed information on state laws and regulations that address pest management in schools. According to BP records, 35 states have regulations or rules that specifically address pesticide use in, near, or around schools [25]. Overall, the major and most consistent problems identified in most of the school policies that currently exist are [25, 26]:

1. problems with communication (getting the information to people who need it);
2. lack of education and training of parents, school administrators, teachers, maintenance staff, and pest management professionals;
3. lack of proper notification and monitoring;
4. lack of implementation and regulation, with no penalties attached to noncompliance with IPM rules;
5. conflicts in IPM policy interpretation; and
6. lack of financing and administrative support for such programs.

Such variation, along with the assortment of state and local regulations, are leading many advocates to call for a standardization of IPM policies with comprehensive federal legislation.

While more than 50 percent of states have IPM policies in place, adherence and enforcement appear to be lax. In New Jersey, for example, the Bureau of Pesticide Operations undertook a small-scale enforcement initiative to evaluate compliance with the School IPM Law that went into effect in 2004. Eighty-four public and private schools in three counties were inspected during the course of a month in 2007. Seventy-four percent of schools in this sample (73% of public schools and 80% of private schools) were found to have major violations, with 7 percent having only minor violations and 19 percent in full compliance. As a result of these findings, the state passed licensing reform mandating more extensive education for pesticide applicators servicing schools. They also increased training and education outreach to inspectors from the local health departments, parents, and teachers [27].

In Texas, where the sufficiency rate of schools with IPM plans on file is 92 percent, the Consumer Protection Division of the Texas Department of Agriculture was able to inspect 70 percent of the 200 schools scheduled for inspection in 2011. Of the schools inspected, only 52.4 percent were found to be in complete compliance, although the nature and severity of the violations were not publicly available [28].

In Massachusetts, the reality of IPM enforcement is not any less discouraging. As in other states, compliance with the regulation is twofold: 1) Every public and private school must submit an IPM plan; and 2) the schools must abide by their plans with regular inspections performed by the Department of Agricultural Resources (MDAR). As of February 2012, 97 percent among the state's 2,867 public and private K-12 schools had achieved compliance with the first requirement [29]. However, the rate of compliance with the second requirement was not an actively maintained statistic. Hundreds of inspection records taken since 2000 are stowed away in paper form. This archaic records system effectively makes an evaluation of the state IPM law quite burdensome. Consequently, the frequency and severity of violations since the law's introduction remain unreported. However, a brief foray into the records by MDAR staff [30] did reveal that in the year 2011, 75 schools were inspected. An annual inspection rate of 3 percent of Massachusetts' nearly 3,000 schools reflects an underpowered policy. Massachusetts' story is not unique; the resources to fully implement state IPM codes are often inadequate and underfunded.

While over 70 percent of states have enacted integrated pest management policies for their schools, many states still lack any legislation or struggle to effectively implement their regulations. In recent years, researchers have investigated ways to strengthen IPM adoption through management strategies and social theory. The Monroe Model, which builds upon and reinforces community engagement, regular communication between stakeholders, and professional recognition and mentoring in a step-by-step process, has proven to be an effective and innovative tool in establishing and sustaining IPM implementation in school districts. An evaluation of 10 school districts in seven states that applied the Monroe Model reported an average reduction of pesticide use of 71 percent over the course of 1-10 years [31]. Furthermore, the model facilitated the diffusion of IPM implementation to neighboring districts—a promising approach to promoting school IPM while federal legislation slowly gains momentum.

IPM LEGISLATION

As the call for federal legislation continues, a recently published report entitled *School IPM 2015: A Strategic Plan for Integrated Pest Management in Schools in the United States* assesses the status of pest management in U.S. school systems and sets out a plan of action to achieve full implementation of IPM in all U.S. schools by 2015 [26]. The development of this strategic plan involved input from a variety of stakeholders representing organized labor, universities, various government agencies, and public/private advocacy organizations across the United States. Participants involved in the development of the plan ranked and identified priorities in four major categories for the optimization of IPM in U.S. schools: regulation, management, research, and education. Among the regulatory priorities, stakeholders ranked and identified increased funding for the enforcement of existing regulations, including compliance by commercial PMPs and businesses providing services to schools as a top priority. Ranked fifth among the top 10 regulatory priorities was to mandate and create minimum standards for school IPM at the federal level, including applicator licensing and a written IPM program through new legislation [26].

In part due to the anti-regulatory climate of the past 10 years, attempts to propose federal legislation for IPM in schools have been unsuccessful. For over 10 years, Beyond Pesticides has led the charge calling for federal legislation to implement IPM in schools. According to BP, the School Environment Protection Act (SEPA) was first introduced by both the U.S. House of Representatives and U.S. Senate in 1999 and then reintroduced in 2001 [32]. BP worked with several legislators in 2001, along with several industry groups to negotiate language that would be accepted by all parties, including the lawn care industry representatives, mosquito control lobbyists, and others. The negotiated bill was attached as an amendment to the No Child Left Behind Act and passed unanimously by the Senate. The Senate voted down the amendment to the education bill by one vote. The same negotiated SEPA amendment was then passed as a part of the Farm Bill in February 2002, but it was later withdrawn due to the House Agriculture Committee's strong opposition and the pesticide industry's silence after previous support [32].

In 2003, the original SEPA was re-introduced by Representatives Rush Holt (D-NJ) and George Miller (D-CA) as part of the Leave No Child Behind Act of 2003; and it was re-introduced in the Senate by Senators Dodd (D-CT) and Kennedy (D-MA) as a part of the same education bill. The SEPA of 2007 (H.R. 3290) was introduced by Representative Holt (D-NJ) and subsequently referred to the Committee on Agriculture during the 110th Congress on August 1, 2007. H.R. 3290 was an amendment to the Federal Insecticide, Fungicide, and Rodenticide Act, and it required the EPA administrator to: 1) establish a National School IPM Advisory System to develop and update uniform standards and criteria for implementing IPM systems in schools; 2) establish a National School IPM Advisory Board; and 3) provide grants to local educational agencies to develop such systems [33]. The bill also prohibited pesticide applications when the school ground or school is in use or occupied and required a 24-hour period between the time an area or room is treated with a pesticide and the time it is used. The bill also prescribed civil penalties for violation of the act and called for the establishment of an IPM trust fund to provide training, education, propagation, and developmental activities under school IPM systems. In part due to industry silence and lack of support, there were no co-sponsors of the bill; and, unfortunately, SEPA 2007 died before making it out of the House Agriculture Committee and ever becoming law.

On December 2, 2009, Representative Holt and 14 co-sponsors introduced what is now considered a "new and improved version" of the School Environment Protection Act (SEPA-HR 4159) that better defines IPM and least toxic pesticides. The new SEPA requires that all schools establish a defined IPM program that emphasizes the use of non-chemical strategies to manage pest problems and the use of least toxic pesticides only as a last resort [34]. The new bill now defines least toxic pesticides as products that are noncarcinogenic; not reproductive, developmental, or nervous system toxicants; and not known as endocrine disruptors—or have not been totally evaluated for their health effects. Under the newly proposed legislation, synthetic fertilizers are prohibited from use on school grounds due to their adverse impact on healthy plants, soils, and turf. There is a provision in the bill to allow the use of a pesticide only in a public health emergency. If indeed there is such a public health emergency that requires pesticide use, parents and guardians of students and the school staff must receive notification of the pesticide application. The legislation also establishes a 12-member National School IPM Advisory Board to develop school IPM standards and a list of allowable least toxic pesticide products with the assistance of a technical advisory panel. Designation of an IPM Coordinator will be required at all local education agencies; and as a part of its existing state cooperative agreement with EPA, each state is required to develop its IPM plan. This legislation would not preempt states or localities with already established IPM policies that exceed the proposed standards [34]. Although in rural school districts pesticides manage to enter the school environment via drift from neighboring farms, passing robust school IPM regulation is a critical step in the effort to limit exposure among students and school workers [5].

The challenges of school IPM policies are multifold but not prohibitive. The enforcement of IPM regulations relies heavily on community involvement from school employees and parents. With state agencies constrained by limited budgets and other resources needed to maintain regular inspections, the burden falls on the community. This, in effect, requires school employees, parents, and students to be educated on their schools' IPM codes. Additionally, IPM practices, while cost-effective in the long run, do require an initial financial expense to get running. The Northeast IPM Center has attempted to mitigate these issues through a competitive grant process to fund IPM projects, with particular emphasis on schools in 13 states. The grants, funded by the U.S. Department of Agriculture, are administered jointly by Pennsylvania State University and Cornell University and aim to develop and evaluate IPM strategies through academic and community partnerships [35].

A WAY FORWARD

When it comes to pesticide exposure and the school environment, our nation's children are the least protected. A federal IPM law is the best way of ensuring that all children in America's schools are adequately protected from exposure to hazardous pesticides used to control pests. Collaborative partnerships—particularly with environmental organizations, school administrators, teachers, parents, parent organizations, labor groups, PMPs, and pest control contractors—must be developed in order to ensure that an effective IPM policy is adopted and implemented. Secondly, financial and administrative support of such a policy must be evident. In addition, in order to achieve compliance with and adherence to an IPM policy, penalties must be assessed for noncompliance and/or incentives must be offered to schools or contractors that adopt and practice sound IPM. Federal legislation is the means for providing consistency in the language of school IPM policies, which is currently lacking. The School Environment Protection Act of 2009 (HR 4159) introduced on December 2, 2009, with 14 co-sponsors, is a positive way forward. A broad coalition of over 25 organizations, including the American Federation of State County and Municipal Employees International (AFSCME), the American Federation of Teachers (AFT), the Center for Environmental Health, California Safe Schools, the Maryland Pesticide Network, the Maine Farmers and Gardeners Association, Osborne Organics, and the Healthy Schools Network, are supporters of SEPA 2009 [36]. A letter-writing and phone campaign was begun to garner additional congressional co-sponsors of the bill. In order for this bill to pass and ever move out of the House Committee on Agriculture, parent groups and organizations around the country should feel that they have a personal stake in protecting children from pesticide-related illnesses and exposure, and they should actively support and advocate for this legislation.

NOTES

1. G. W. Nalyanya et al., "German Cockroach Allergen Levels in North Carolina Schools: Comparison of Integrated Pest Management and Conventional Cockroach Control," *Journal of Medical Entomology* 46(3) (2009): 420-427.
2. J. N. Parker, "Reducing Asthma Triggers in Schools: Recommendations for Effective Policies, Regulations, and Legislation," *New Solutions: A Journal of Environmental and Occupational Health Policy* 16(1) (2006): 87-105.
3. B. L. Brenner et al., "Integrated Pest Management in an Urban Community: A Successful Partnership for Prevention," *Environmental Health Perspectives* 111(13) (2003): 1649-1653.
4. Maryland Pesticide Network, *Are We Passing the Grade? Assessing MD Schools' Compliance with IPM In-Schools Law: A Report by the Maryland Pesticide Network*, September 2004.
5. W. Alarcon, G. Calvert, and J. Blondell, "Acute Illnesses Associated with Pesticide Exposure at Schools," *Journal of American Medical Association* 294(4) (2005): 455-465.
6. C. Piper and K. Owens, "Are Schools Making the Grade? School Districts Nationwide Adopt Safer Pest Management Policies," *Pesticides and You, Beyond Pesticides/ National Coalition against the Misuse of Pesticides* 22(3) (2002): 11-20.
7. Jonathan Kaplan, Sandra Marquardt, and Wendy Barber (CALPIRG Charitable Trust), *Failing Health: Pesticide Use in California Schools* (Californians for Pesticide Reform, 1998).
8. California Department of Pesticide Regulation, "The Healthy Schools Act: What's Mandatory? What's Voluntary?," http://apps.cdpr.ca.gov/schoolipm/school_ipm_law/34_HSA_Mand.cfm?crumbs_list=#MandatoryDetails (accessed on June 27, 2012).
9. Pesticide Regulation Section of the Maryland Department of Agriculture, *Integrated Pest Management in Schools: IPM Training Manual,* YEAR, http://www.mda.state.md.us/pdf/ipmmanua.pdf (accessed June 27, 2012).
10. C. A. Geiger and D. H. Tootelian, "Healthy Schools Act Spurs Integrated Pest Management in California Public Schools," *California Agriculture* 59(4) (2005): 235-241.
11. Western Region School IPM Implementation Assessment Work Group, *Inventory of School IPM Programs: State Narratives*, 2008.
12. P. L. Nixon and C. Clark, *School IPM Implementation in Illinois Final Grant Report* (Urbana, IL: University of Illinois Extension, 2007).
13. Californians for Alternatives to Toxics, *Are Our Schools Flunking Out? A Mid-Term Report Card on Chemical Pest Management*, 2004.
14. A. E. Brown and J. Z. Schmidt, "Response to Pre-notification of Pesticide Application in a Public School System," *Journal of Pesticide Education* 2 (2000): 1-14.
15. North Carolina State University, *Integrated Pest Management in North Carolina Schools: A Sample of School Districts That Have Implemented IPM Programs*, 2007, http://schoolipm.nscu.edu/documents/schools.pdf (accessed August 11, 2009).
16. G. W. Nalyanya et al., "Practices and Perceptions of School Integrated Pest Management by North Carolina Pest-Management Professional," *Journal of Agricultural Urban Entomology* 22(3,4) (2005): 203-215.

17. West Virginia Department of Agriculture, *Title 61 Legislative Rules, Integrated Pest Management Programs in Schools and Day Care Centers, Series 12J*, 1996.
18. Maryland Department of Agriculture, Title 15, Subtitle 05, Pesticide Use Control, Chapter 2: Integrated Pest Management and Notification of Pesticide Use in a Public School Building or on School Grounds, 1999.
19. North Carolina Department of Agriculture, Structural Pest Control Regulations for North Carolina, Section.0300, Licensing and Certification, Statutory Authority G-S, 106-65.29, 1977.
20. L. Weiss and S. Moran, *Pest Control Practices in Oregon Public Schools* (Portland, OR: Oregon Environmental Council, 2005).
21. Laura Braband, Edward Horn, and Laura Sahr, *Pest Management Practices A Survey of Public School Districts in New York State*, NYS IPM Number 613, NYSAES, Geneva, NY, 2002.
22. S. S. Addiss et al., *Pest Control Practices in Connecticut Public Schools* (North Haven, CT: Environment and Human Health, Inc., 1999).
23. G. W. Nalyanya and S. Lilley, *Pest Control Practices in North Carolina Public Schools* (Raleigh, NC: North Carolina State University IPM Center, College of Agriculture and Life Sciences, 2002).
24. Michael H. Surgan, Judith Enck, and Alice Yu, *Pesticide Use at New York Schools: Reducing the Risk, Environmental Protection Bureau*, Office of the Attorney General, New York, 2000.
25. Beyond Pesticides, "State and Local School Pesticide Policies," http://www.beyond pesticides.org/schools/schoolpolicies/index.htm (accessed September 7, 2009).
26. T. A. Green and D. H. Gouge (eds.), *School IPM 2015: A Strategic Plan for Integrated Pest Management in Schools in the United States*, The IPM Institute and Department of Entomology, University of Arizona, February 25, 2009.
27. New Jersey Department of Environmental Protection, Bureau of Enforcement & Compliance Services, *Fiscal Year 2008 Compliance & Enforcement Highlights Report*, 2008, http://www.nj.gov/dep/enforcement/cehighlightsfy2008.pdf (accessed on June 27, 2012).
28. M. E. Merchant, Texas A&M Agrilife Extension, "School Integrated Pest Management/ Structural Pest Control Service Winter Update," http://schoolipm.tamu.edu/2012/ 01/30/structural-pest-control-service-winter-update (accessed April 16, 2012).
29. T. Battle, Massachusetts Department of Agricultural Resources, "Compliance Rates for IPM Plan Development and Submission as of August 16, 2011," http://massnrc.org/ipm/news/compliance_rates.html (accessed on June 27, 2012).
30. Massachusetts Department of Agricultural Resources staff, personal communication, May 1, 2012.
31. D. H. Gouge, M. L. Lame, and J. L. Snyder, "Use of an Implementation Model and Diffusion Process for Establishing Integrated Pest Management in Arizona Schools," *American Entomologist* 52(3) (2006): 190-196.
32. Beyond Pesticides, "Previous Efforts to Pass SEPA," http://www.beyondpesticides. org/schools/sepa/index.htm (accessed November 12, 2009).
33. Civic Impulse, LLC, "Govtrack.us / HR 3290(110th): School Environment Protection Act of 2007," http://www.govtrack.us/congress/bill.xpd?bill=h110-3290 (accessed September 7, 2009).

34. Beyond Pesticides, *Children, Pesticides, and Schools: School Environment Protection Act of 2009*, http:/www.beyondpesticides.org/schools/sepa/SEPA2009bill summary.pdf (accessed December 4, 2009).
35. Northeastern IPM Center, "Northeast Regional IPM Competitive Grants," http://www.northeastipm.org/grant-programs/ipm-center-grants/northeast-regional-ipm-competitive-grants/ (accessed June 27, 2012).
36. Beyond Pesticides, *SEPA List of Supporters*, http://www.beyondpesticides.org/schools/sepa/SEPA2009supporters.pdf (accessed December 4, 2009).

CHAPTER 12

Reducing Asthma Triggers in Schools: Recommendations for Effective Policies, Regulations, and Legislation*

Joan N. Parker

According to the National Center for Health Statistics, 24.6 million Americans surveyed in 2009 reported having been diagnosed with asthma. Children have been severely affected: asthma is the most common chronic childhood disease and one of the leading causes of school absenteeism. A survey conducted by The National Association of School Nurses found that asthma is more disruptive of school routines than any other chronic condition. Asthma is also common among teachers, an indication that the school building environment may be associated with asthma prevalence in all occupants of school buildings.

Children are particularly sensitive to environmental pollutants, which are more concentrated in indoor air environments than in outdoor environments. Schools are a significant source of indoor air pollutants, and children spend a large portion of their lives in these buildings. Yet little research has been conducted that addresses the causal relationship between asthma and specific levels of indoor pollutants including mold, fungi, and bacteria.

By and large, indoor air quality is not controlled in schools in a way that minimizes exposures that cause or aggravate asthma. While there are few laws that specifically limit indoor air pollutants in schools, there are several laws that

*This chapter was originally written in 2005 as a report for the Asthma Regional Council of New England, a coalition of public agencies, private organizations, and researchers across working to tackle environmental and clinical aspects of pediatric and adult asthma. The ARC is a program of Health Resources in Action. The report was updated in 2012.

outline or mandate practices that can effectively control exposures. This chapter provides concise recommendations for laws and regulations to control and prevent indoor air quality problems, with the goal of reducing the occurrence and severity of asthma and other respiratory diseases. A snapshot summarizing these recommendations appears at the end of the chapter.

METHODOLOGY

Indoor air quality laws and regulations for schools were reviewed in 2005 to determine which states provide good models for protecting students and staff. No state had an ideal regulatory package. Therefore, what is presented here is a compilation of recommendations based on the best laws in several states at the time. These recommendations come mainly from those states with the best overall structures, but certain aspects of other states' laws have been incorporated if they appeared to be particularly innovative, protective, or synergistic with the laws from the model states. While most of the recommendations presented here are based on existing laws, some are based on policies and practices that have been shown to be effective, but are not currently required by law.

The recommendations are aimed at prevention and control of asthma, but they also recognize that it is beneficial to consider other health effects caused by exposure to indoor air pollutants, such as allergic reactions, including skin and eye irritation, and other respiratory conditions, including hypersensitivity pneumonitis and reactive airway disease. These conditions may indicate exposures that also have the potential to cause or aggravate asthma. Therefore, the recommendations are not limited to controls that only prevent exposure to known asthmagens.

In addition, it is important to expand the generally accepted view that mold and other microbiologicals are the only indoor air pollutants in schools responsible for causing or aggravating asthma. Other potential causes include volatile organic compounds, such as solvents in cleaning and art supplies, and particulate matter, such as diesel exhaust, dust, and other byproducts of construction and renovation work.

The recommendations that follow are broken down into the main technical areas that relate to minimizing indoor air pollution in schools. These areas are:

1. maintenance of buildings;
2. ventilation systems;
3. design, new construction, and renovation; and
4. chemicals and other materials, including their purchase, storage, disposal, and safe use.

For each of these areas, the most important elements that address asthma are summarized, and sample language from state laws is quoted or cited. For an excellent comprehensive review of all states' indoor air quality laws, see the Environmental Law Institute's research report, *Building Healthy, High Performance*

Schools: A Review of Selected State and Local Initiatives [1]. In addition, the National Association of State Boards of Education (NASBE) has released an on-line publication, *Issue Brief: Summary and Analysis of State Policies on Asthma Education, Medications, and Triggers* [2]. This 20-page issue brief synthesizes current, as of 2005, state policies addressing various asthma-related topics, which NASBE has collected in its state school health policy database. Among the topics addressed are asthma education, identification of students with asthma, administration of medications by school staff, self-administration of medications, tobacco-free schools, air quality, pest control, and other environmental health policies.

The recommendations presented here differ from the documents cited above in that they not only reference model laws, but also include suggestions for improving upon those laws. In making these recommendations, consideration has been given to cost-effectiveness, to long-range benefits, and to avoiding conflict with existing laws or standards for environments other than schools.

RECOMMENDATIONS

Ventilation Systems

Any indoor air quality law must require that schools adhere to minimum ventilation standards. The most efficient way to prevent the buildup of indoor air pollutants, apart from complete source elimination, is through effective ventilation. A good ventilation system must function properly, according to design specifications, and must comply with minimum standards established by state building codes or, in this case, laws designed to reduce exposure to asthmagens and other irritants in schools.

Many state laws require compliance with the specifications of Standard 62, titled "Ventilation for Acceptable Indoor Air Quality,"[3] which is prepared and routinely updated by the American Society for Heating, Refrigeration, and Air Conditioning Engineers, Inc. (ASHRAE). This standard is not a legal requirement, but it can be incorporated into law. The state of Maine, for example, requires that Standard 62 be applied to all buildings occupied by state employees [4]. This requirement should be altered to include and to apply specifically to all school buildings. In addition, the law should make clear that the schools' ventilation systems must comply with the ASHRAE standard that is or was current at the time the ventilation system was installed or renovated.

Minnesota goes further and requires certification that, for any new or extensively renovated facility, the heating, ventilation, and air conditioning (HVAC) system "will meet or exceed code standards; will provide for the monitoring of outdoor airflow and total airflow of ventilation systems; and will provide an indoor air quality filtration system . . ." that meets the most updated standard [5].

What is crucial, however, is that certain specific minimum standards for ventilation be clearly established. For example, ASHRAE Standard 62.1 for classrooms with children ages 5 through 8 specifies that each school should provide a minimum of 10 cubic feet per minute of outside air for each person [3]. More should be provided in certain areas, such as gyms, rest rooms, lockers, and kitchens, where additional dilution is important [3]. The air supplied to each occupant should consist of 25 percent outside air [6]. Recirculating more than 75 percent of the total air can result in an excessive build-up of any contaminants present in the environment.

The total amount of incoming air available per person is as important as the proportion of fresh, outside air. Increasing the total amount of incoming air increases the rate of removal of contaminants through the room's exhaust system. For maximum dilation, each room or area should undergo 10 full air changes per hour [7].

HVAC or related systems should be able to provide a range of 30 to 60 percent relative humidity [8]. Levels greater than 70 percent are conducive to microbial growth and levels less than 30 percent are drying and may increase sensitivity to irritants in the air.

HVAC systems should be operated continuously during all hours of occupation so that before- and after-school activities don't take place in unhealthy environments. Most of the states recognize that some exceptions to this requirement will be necessary, and that these should be specified. For example, most states drop the requirement for ventilation during scheduled maintenance and emergency repairs.

Ventilation systems should be routinely inspected to ensure proper functioning and to facilitate maintenance, which is covered in another section of this report. California's standards for workplaces require that HVAC systems be inspected at least annually and that inspections and maintenance of the HVAC system be documented in writing, listing the name of the individual inspecting and/or maintaining the system, the date of the inspection and/or maintenance, and the specific findings and actions taken. The state further requires that the records be kept for at least five years and that they be available to employees upon request [9].

To further increase the effectiveness of this requirement, the law should reference a straightforward checklist for inspecting the HVAC system. Minnesota has developed an operations and maintenance manual for such a purpose [10].

In addition to general ventilation systems, which do no more than dilute contaminants in the air, local exhaust systems are necessary to remove recognized chemicals and toxins in certain areas of known risk. Examples of areas that should be equipped with systems to remove hazardous gases and particulates without recirculation of air include chemistry and biology labs, art classrooms and facilities, auto-body and mechanical shops, woodworking and metalworking shops, and areas in which cleaning and maintenance products are stored. Auto-body shops are particularly hazardous because of their use of isocyanates, which can aggravate existing asthma and can cause asthma in individuals with no history of the disease. An indoor air quality law should reference or include the specifications contained in workplace standards on local exhaust ventilation. California's general industry safety orders that cover dusts, fumes, mists, vapors, and gases serve as a good reference [11].

Fume hoods are a form of local exhaust ventilation and should, at a minimum, conform to the most recent version of the American National Standard for Laboratory Ventilation [12]. Testing methods to determine compliance should follow the ASHRAE Method of Testing Performance of Laboratory Fume Hoods [13]. Fume hoods should be on at all times and should never be used to store hazardous or toxic chemicals.

The preceding recommendations are of a technical nature, but some common-sense recommendations are also in order. For example, it is crucial that the outside air intakes for ventilation systems be located away from any possible contaminants, such as parking lots, areas where fuel-burning equipment is operated, trash containers, outdoor painting applications, or exhaust from other areas within the building, such as cafeterias, laboratories, janitors' closets, and trade shops [14]. In addition, all vents that exhaust air from hazardous areas should be located so that the contaminated air does not re-enter the building or expose students or school personnel when they are outside the building. To ensure the effectiveness of the above recommendations, the system should be regularly inspected, repaired, maintained, and updated.

Maintenance

A well-designed and properly functioning ventilation system is critically dependent upon effective maintenance. In addition, maintenance and cleaning can significantly reduce the opportunities for exposure to respiratory hazards. A conscientious *routine maintenance* program will decrease the need for *emergency maintenance* and repairs, thereby reducing the duration of exposure and eliminating unanticipated costs for such emergency work.

Most states require maintenance of *ventilation systems* in school buildings, but often fail to require routine maintenance that also addresses the *broader areas*, such as proper and frequent cleaning of buildings, which can prevent or reduce indoor air quality problems. Many laws also fail to specify a schedule or particular criteria for such maintenance.

Vermont law requires that a model policy be implemented, to include the "compilation of a recommended maintenance schedule and checklist for the school, summarizing when and how maintenance of heating and ventilation systems should occur" [15]. The Vermont law could be improved by listing the specific criteria for maintenance and schedules, perhaps by referencing and requiring compliance with ASHRAE's Standard 62 or the EPA's Tools for Schools [3, 16]. This section of the law should clarify whether or not the maintenance is mandatory and should clearly include all phases of maintenance in addition to the HVAC system.

Connecticut law is broader and does not limit maintenance to the HVAC system. It requires that "Each local or regional board of education . . . shall undertake maintenance of its facilities" and "shall adopt and implement an indoor air quality program that provides for ongoing maintenance and facility reviews necessary for the maintenance and improvement of the indoor air quality in its facilities . . ." [17, 18]. This law, like the Vermont law, fails to include specific schedules and criteria for maintenance, but it does require that HVAC systems be "maintained . . . in accordance with the prevailing maintenance standards, such as Standard 62, at the time of installation or renovation of such system" [19]. Standard 62 does recommend maintenance schedules [3]. The shortcoming of this section is that it addresses only maintenance *schedules* that relate to the HVAC system. The law should reference a standard that includes all phases of maintenance, as does the EPA's Tools for Schools [16].

Maintenance procedures and schedules should address the day-to-day cleaning of classrooms, offices, common spaces, personal service rooms, storerooms, and utility areas. As per California's General Industry Safety Orders, cleaning should be done with the following considerations [20]:

- Wet or damp mopping is the ideal way to clean floors without increasing the amount of suspended particulate matter in the air.
- Vacuuming is always preferable to dry sweeping and should be done using a high-efficiency particulate air (HEPA) filtration machine.
- The choice of cleaning materials should take into consideration their toxicity and potential to cause respiratory problems.
- Whenever possible, cleaning should be done when the area is not occupied, and large cleaning projects should be done in areas that are sealed off from occupied areas.

In addition to specifying maintenance procedures, a good law will recommend appropriate criteria for responding to reports of health problems or other conditions that may be related to indoor air quality. The model school environmental management plan required by Vermont law must include "mechanisms to resolve hazardous chemical exposure and indoor air quality problems as they occur . . . " [21].

A thorough and effective maintenance program can be implemented by following the recommendations contained within EPA's Tools for Schools program [16]. EPA has more specific recommendations for response to and cleanup of mold and moisture [22]. These programs should be integrated into indoor air quality laws.

Another good reference for maintenance is the "checklist for schools," developed by the Massachusetts Multi-Agency Task Force on Schools [23].

A very important means of reducing exposure to microbial contaminants (i.e., mold, mildew, fungus, bacteria) is ensuring that carpets that become wet be dried within 24 hours. Wet carpets provide an ideal growth medium for mold and mildew, and attempts at drying them after they have been wet for more than 24 hours are rarely successful. Wet carpets and rugs should be disposed of after one day [24].

Appropriate laws that specify maintenance procedures and schedules cannot be effective unless maintenance personnel are appropriately trained to carry out their duties. Such training is essential, in particular, when an emergency arises that requires immediate attention.

Vermont law requires that "The commissioners of health and of buildings and general services, education and health, with help from the secretary of the agency of natural resources when appropriate, shall . . . organize school environmental health training workshop[s] for school environmental health coordinators and school administrators, and an annual training for school maintenance and custodial staff . . ." [25].

Connecticut law requires that training of maintenance personnel be reviewed during inspections, which must be conducted every five years, and those inspections are limited to new construction and buildings renovated after January 2, 2003 [26]. Both the Connecticut and Vermont laws could be improved by providing criteria for the training; the Connecticut law could be improved by requiring the training for maintenance staff in all buildings, and by making the training mandatory, rather than simply making it a subject for inspection.

Chemicals and Products: How to Choose, Store, and Use

One of the reasons that ventilation and maintenance are so critical in ensuring a healthy environment is the ubiquity of hazardous materials encountered inside buildings. Sources include cleaning and maintenance products; paints and other coatings; furnishings; trade shops; building materials; and maintenance, repair, and renovation projects. A sufficient quantity of air and good filtration of the air entering the building will significantly reduce pollutants from the outside. To aid in reducing exposures originating indoors, however, it is crucial to eliminate or significantly reduce the concentration of those materials that can cause or aggravate asthma.

Rhode Island has passed model indoor air quality legislation, known as the Rules and Regulations for School Health Programs, amended October 2003, which includes a comprehensive list of approximately 500 chemicals that may not be purchased or used in schools [27]. Their regulations also specify a general chemical hygiene program for schools. Adding a list of specific nontoxic or low toxicity building materials would further strengthen these regulations. The Massachusetts Executive Office of Environmental Affairs has developed a list of Environmentally Preferable Products for schools and municipalities, many of which have been reviewed for health effects [28].

In 2005, the state of Maine passed *An Act to Protect Children from Toxic Chemicals in Schools*, which funds a chemical clean-out program through a tax on certain pesticides. The state's Departments of Environmental Protection and Education were charged with working together to implement the plan. The program is now referred to as "Hazardous Chemicals in our Schools" [29].

Some states rely upon nongovernmental organizations for recommendations regarding chemicals and materials to use or avoid as a means of reducing environmental impact [30, 31]. However, few states focus strictly on health criteria, and fewer still on respiratory health criteria, to comprehensively regulate the purchase or use of chemicals or other materials.

Federal and state "right-to-know" laws impose requirements for *providing information* about certain hazardous chemicals, but these laws do not *prohibit the use* of such materials [32, 33]. Respiratory hazards are not specifically addressed in most of these laws. For example, the Massachusetts Right-to-Know Law regulates the information that is released about certain categories of hazardous chemicals more stringently than others, but the law does not regard respiratory hazards as a category that warrants special restriction.

Outright prohibition of the use of toxic materials is rare. Most laws that ban specific materials are federal laws, such as those that ban asbestos, lead, and mercury. The ban that had the greatest potential to influence respiratory health in schools was the 1982 ban on urea-formaldehyde foam insulation. The ban was lifted, however, shortly after it was issued [34].

Workplace health and safety laws, which are based on human health, do not prohibit the use of materials, but they do limit the concentrations to which workers may be exposed. However, these limits are often not sufficiently protective of healthy, self-selected working populations, much less the more vulnerable population of children, particularly those with respiratory illness. There is limited information about the concentrations of chemicals or other hazardous materials that may cause or aggravate asthma. In addition, many chemicals used or manufactured in the workplace are not regulated at all. For these reasons, it is critical to limit exposure to respiratory hazards to the extent possible.

A law designed to effectively reduce the risk of asthma should address:

- materials whose use must be limited to certain concentration levels;
- materials whose use is prohibited;
- materials that can be used or stored only under specified conditions;
- materials that are recommended for specific purposes; and
- conditions under which certain materials cannot be used.

The EPA Tools for Schools is a document that provides extensive guidance on indoor air quality in schools, including how to manage chemical use and disposal [16]. More specific guidance on managing chemicals already in use in schools is provided in a document assembled by an environmental consultant for the Burlington, Massachusetts, Health Department [35]. These guidelines should be incorporated by reference, as recommended under the section on Maintenance.

Rhode Island's law provides a good example for reducing exposures to chemical hazards. Following are additional elements that can be incorporated into law to more specifically reduce exposures to chemicals and products that may cause or aggravate asthma and other respiratory conditions.

- Use the least toxic and most easily maintained flooring. Consult the Asthma Regional Council of New England's guide to the purchase and use of healthy flooring [36].
- If carpeting must be used, consult the CRI Indoor Air Quality Green Label Plus Program for testing results on the components of the carpet, adhesive, and pad [37].
- Use the least toxic paints, sealants, coatings and adhesives, preferably those that are listed as "low VOC" or "zero VOC." (Particularly avoid acid-cured wood floor finishes.)
- Purchase only paints that do not contain formaldehyde and that do not generate formaldehyde while they are drying [38].
- Purchase only furnishings and other building materials, such as chip board, that do not contain or generate formaldehyde.
- Use building materials for indoor surfaces that are non-porous, making them easier to clean and less likely to serve as a medium for the growth of mold, bacteria, and fungus.
- Purchase products without fragrances or other respiratory irritants.
- Do not use ozone generators or air purifiers that emit ozone.
- Reduce exposure to cockroaches and other insects that can cause or aggravate asthma, but ensure that the use of pesticides is a last resort and that, where used, they are applied under an integrated pest management system. A good example of such a system was developed by the California School Integrated Pest Management Program [39]. Massachusetts has one of the most restrictive laws addressing pesticide use in schools and in day-care centers [40].
- Eliminate or control exposure to animals in classrooms and other areas of schools.
- Prohibit smoking of any materials in school buildings and on school grounds.
- Do not purchase or use latex gloves or other latex products that may cause or aggravate asthma.
- Do not purchase products without first reviewing and giving preference to those that are approved by Green Seal and Massachusetts' Environmentally Preferable Products Procurement Program [41, 42].
- Do not purchase materials that contain or emit isocyanates or urethanes.
- Complete a regular inventory of stored chemicals and properly dispose of those no longer used, needed, or safe.

Regardless of the progress any school may make in reducing the number of materials that may cause or aggravate asthma, it is essential that staff, students, and their parents have full knowledge of the actual exposures that may be encountered at school. For this reason, states that do not have their own right-to-know laws should incorporate the federal Hazard Communication Standard or another state's right-to-know law into a similar law of their own.[1] Some states have community right-to-know laws that may fill the gap. The federal Hazard Communication Standard applies only to private-sector employees, but its requirements in that sector can be applied by incorporating them into state law. Rhode Island did this with respect to its chemical hygiene plan for schools [27].

Vermont law requires the commissioner of education to distribute to all public schools a "model environmental health management plan" which "provides suggestions for communicating school environmental health status to building occupants and parents . . ." [21]. This requirement could be strengthened by specifying the criteria and timelines for communicating hazards and by making such communication mandatory.

Design, Construction, and Renovation

Many of the common indoor air quality problems can be prevented by prudent design of new construction and major renovation. Good design is cost-effective in that it can significantly reduce the cost of subsequent repairs and renovation. Laws should include a list of materials that are known or suspected to cause or aggravate respiratory problems and prohibit their use in new or renovated school buildings. Ventilation and cooling systems have a critical effect on subsequent indoor air quality. The recommendations contained in the previous sections should serve as standards for design and renovation.

Design of new or renovated schools should reflect the most stringent standards at the time of construction. For example, some ventilation designs may *allow* operation that complies with these standards, but the same designs may not *prevent* operation that falls outside the standards. A case in point is the ventilation system design that provides a variable volume of outside air, determined by the outdoor temperature. In an effort to reduce costs for cooling or heating, outside air that is above or below certain temperatures will be limited, and may be limited to fall below the standard set by building code or non-mandatory criteria. New designs should ensure that the reduction of outside air does not allow the quantity to fall below the minimum criteria.

Massachusetts has been very successful in devising criteria for new construction and the extensive renovation of school facilities. Schools engaging in such construction should refer to the work of the Massachusetts Technology Park

[1]The federal OSHA Hazard Communication Standard does not apply to public-sector employers.

Collaborative (MTC), a quasi-governmental agency that has supported the drafting of a manual for construction of "high performance schools" [43]. Such schools are those that meet strict criteria related to sustainability, energy conservation, and environment, including the indoor environment. These criteria are based on those developed by California's Collaborative for High Performance Schools.

A crucial issue covered in the manual is how to address indoor air quality during construction and renovation projects. Some states, including Massachusetts and Connecticut, have required the use of the Sheet Metal and Air Conditioning Contractors National Association (SMACNA) *IAQ Guidelines for Occupied Buildings under Construction* [44]. Adherence to these guidelines should be a condition of all school construction projects. All reputable contractors will have access to the SMACNA guidelines. These guidelines list recommendations to reduce exposures, including the following:

- Perform as much of the work as possible when the building is not occupied.
- Keep building occupants as far from the construction as possible.
- Install temporary barriers and ensure that the ventilation system is not drawing any pollutants to occupied areas (create positive pressure in those areas).
- Use methods, such as wet methods, that will reduce the concentration of airborne pollutants.

A valuable guide for construction planning and practices that reduce the chance of subsequent health problems is the EPA's Tools for Schools manual on indoor air quality design [45]. The salient recommendations for construction planning include:

- Incorporate indoor air quality goals into the bid and construction documents.
- Require the development and use of an indoor air quality management plan.
- Ensure that all members of the project team are familiar with indoor air quality issues and have defined their responsibilities to address those issues.
- Require contractors to provide information on any product substitutions.

Recommendations for safer construction practices include:

- Keep building materials dry to prevent microbial growth.
- Dry water-damaged materials as soon as possible.
- Clean spills of toxic or irritant materials immediately.
- Seal unnecessary openings.
- Temporarily seal ductwork to prevent contamination during construction (ensuring, however, that workers are provided a safe environment).

Many practices that are crucial for healthy design, construction, and renovation are required as a contingency for funding. As illustrated in the section of this report on funding, many states will not accept bids for contracts unless the proposal incorporates standard practices that optimize indoor air quality.

OVERALL POLICIES TO SUPPORT HEALTHY SCHOOLS

The following sections—assessment, funding, and implementation—address the policies necessary to support the technical recommendations presented in the previous sections. These policies are all interrelated. Assessment of indoor air quality allows schools to carry out the technical recommendations and allows authorities, such as the state department of education or the legislature, to evaluate a school's implementation of state-based laws and mandates. Funding for repairs and renovations is often contingent upon appropriate implementation of those laws and mandates, and the need for funding cannot be determined without a thorough and accurate assessment of the buildings.

Assessment

In order to establish appropriate measures to reduce indoor air pollutants, it is essential to determine the needs within each building. Such a determination requires a thorough assessment of at least:

- the ventilation and cooling systems;
- the chemicals and materials in use or in storage in and around the school;
- the condition of the roof and building envelope;
- the condition of ceilings, walls, floors, and carpets, with special attention to moisture and particulate matter;
- the condition of horizontal surfaces, with regard to dirt and dust;
- the condition of porous materials, such as drapes, furniture and partitions;
- the presence of insects, feathered or furry animals; and
- the schedule, frequency, and effectiveness of maintenance.

Connecticut law requires an inspection and evaluation of the indoor air quality in all school buildings "constructed, extended, renovated or replaced on or after January 1, 2003" [46]. The evaluation must be completed every five years and must cover a broad range of potential sources of indoor air quality problems, such as:

- HVAC systems;
- exposure to airborne microbiological particles, such as fungi, mold, and bacteria;
- the presence of hazardous substances;
- moisture incursion; and
- training of building staff.

The law references the EPA Tools for Schools, a resource that contains several checklists for evaluating indoor air quality in schools [45].

The Connecticut law could be strengthened by extending it to all schools, instead of limiting its coverage to recently constructed or renovated buildings, given that some of the worst ventilation conditions can be found in older buildings.

Connecticut requires an assessment of newer or renovated buildings only once every five years. Maine law, however, requires an annual inspection of the HVAC system, but the inspection is not as broad as that called for by the Connecticut law [47]. Maine law also requires the correction of any HVAC problems identified during the inspection, but does not specify a time period for such correction. Both states require that records of the inspection be maintained, which is critical for evaluating progress and for providing information about past exposures.

Most states depend upon individuals employed by or contracted by the department of education to address indoor air quality issues. In Maine, however, the Division of Safety and Environmental Services, within the Bureau of General Services, provides indoor air quality assessment for public schools.

It can be difficult in some cases to reach agreement about the air quality in an environment, especially if funding for remediation is dependent upon a substantiated need. In Connecticut, if a standard does not exist to dictate how to address the specific conditions, the state may call in outside consultants to evaluate whether or not the indoor air quality is adequate. The University of Connecticut is specifically referenced in the legislation as an example of a source of expert consultants [46].

Funding

An effective means of incorporating good indoor air quality practices into school renovation or construction projects is to require that bidders include in their proposals provisions for minimizing or eliminating health hazards potentially associated with the work. Bidders should also be required to submit a detailed assessment of the status of the indoor air quality in buildings to be renovated.

Improvements to indoor air quality should receive priority status for funding. Maine has established a School Revolving Renovation Fund, which assigns first priority for certain projects, including improving indoor air quality in school buildings [48].

Several states make approval of school building projects contingent upon certain conditions, such as Connecticut's requirement that plans for the construction, renovation, or replacement of a school building include the following: 1) adherence to the SMACNA guidelines to ensure good indoor air quality in occupied buildings under construction; 2) roof construction specifications that minimize the potential for water damage; and 3) indoor air quality training for building maintenance staff [19].

Minnesota and Massachusetts require that state agencies planning major construction or renovations undergo an environmental impact statement (EIS). The local school department may not approve the project until the EIS is reviewed [49]. In Massachusetts, the assessment must conform to ASTM Phase I standards

[50]. A Phase II assessment, which requires actual testing, must be conducted based on the Phase I assessment.

Implementation, Oversight, and Enforcement

Most states designate responsibility for indoor air quality to local or regional school districts or boards of education. To ensure adherence to legal or mandated standards, many laws require that reports of the status of indoor air quality be submitted to the state commissioner of education or to the state legislature. Connecticut, for example, requires that the boards of education "report annually to the Commissioner of Education on the condition of its facilities and the action taken to implement its long-term school building program and indoor air quality" [18]. Maine convened a task force to establish and implement the state's standards for indoor air quality in schools [51]. One of the functions of the task force was "to provide adequate state oversight so that indoor air quality standards for school facilities may be enforced" [51].

Effective compliance with indoor air quality standards is essential, not only for protecting the health of students and staff, but for determining whether or not the standards themselves are sufficiently protective.

There are very few states with laws that contain true enforcement, which makes it difficult to ensure accountability on the part of the agencies responsible for indoor air quality in schools. Maine's law does contain enforcement language, making the school administrative unit responsible for correcting potentially hazardous conditions and holding the unit liable for penalties [52].

As illustrated in the previous section, many states have tied funding to compliance with indoor air quality standards. Rhode Island has done the same, but rather than making prospective funding contingent upon the promise of compliance, the law imposes a penalty for noncompliance in the form of withholding public money that has been apportioned to the city or town [53].

Rhode Island has written some broad language to protect the health and safety of students and staff in its schools. In addition to creating an extensive list of chemicals and materials prohibited in schools, the state has extended OSHA standards to students—standards that generally cover only employees [54].

The age and deteriorating conditions of many schools, the lack of good information about potential health hazards and their control, the high cost of remediating unhealthy conditions, and the dearth of funds for education and capital improvements all contribute to a problem that cannot be easily resolved. While compliance can be difficult and expensive, even with some of the minimal standards, enforcement may be necessary to focus the attention of the accountable entities on creative solutions to a growing problem.

CONCLUSION

School buildings are environments where children not only learn, but where they spend a good portion of their daily lives. School buildings are also environments where the air quality is often poor and where asthma rates are high. There are solutions to these problems, which can be accomplished through adhering to appropriate laws, regulations, and recommendations to improve the air quality in schools.

Some effective national advocacy organizations that are involved in promoting healthy school environments include the:

- National Council for Occupational Safety and Health, which has a list of state COSH chapters (see http://www.coshnetwork.org/COSHGroupsList));
- American Lung Association (ALA), which has a list of state affiliates (see www.lungusa.org/asthma/); and
- National Healthy Schools Network (see http://www.healthyschools.org/index.html).

These organizations can provide assistance in developing strategies and policies to promote healthy schools. School administrators and educators can play an important role in protecting the health of students and staff by becoming familiar with the air quality issues in their schools. They can respond to those issues through thoughtful implementation of the recommendations contained in this report. Often, however, consistent and timely changes must be effected by passing, implementing, and complying with laws and regulations. This report summarizes the best state laws and makes recommendations to minimize conditions that can cause or exacerbate asthma among all school occupants.

Reducing Asthma Triggers in Schools: Summary Recommendations for Effective Policies, Regulations, and Legislation

Ventilation

- At a minimum, comply with the air supply specifications contained in ASHRAE Standard 62, with updates to reflect changes in the standard.
- Provide a minimum of 20 cubic feet per minute of outside air for each occupant, with a greater quantity of air in areas that require more dilution.
- Provide a minimum of 25 percent outside air.
- Provide a minimum of 10 air changes per hour.
- Develop/reference a checklist for inspecting and trouble-shooting the HVAC system.

- Use/install local exhaust ventilation for areas where the use or storage of hazardous materials prevents dependence on dilution ventilation for control of hazards.
- Locate outside air intakes away from any potential sources of contamination.

Maintenance

- Develop/use a standardized maintenance program for the HVAC system and implement it on a regular basis.
- Develop and implement a routine maintenance program, emphasizing cleaning of occupied areas, using methods that minimize particulates in the air.
- Develop and implement a protocol for water damage, including inspection criteria and schedules, immediate response, and remediation.
- Record and maintain details of maintenance activities.
- Develop and implement a protocol for responding to reports of health problems or conditions that may be related to indoor air quality.
- Develop, implement, and document training for maintenance personnel.

Chemicals and products

- Compile a list of chemicals and potentially hazardous materials in use or in storage in all school buildings.
- Develop a protocol for managing and disposing of materials that are hazardous, out of date, or no longer used.
- Develop a list of materials that are not to be used or stored in any school building, on the basis of health, safety, or environmental concerns.
- Use the least toxic materials and develop concentration limits.

Design, construction, and renovation

- Design, construction, and renovation should reflect the most stringent standards at the time of the work.
- Comply with Collaborative for High Performance Schools (CHPS) standards in the design of schools.
- Use Sheet Metal and Air Conditioning Contractors National Association (SMACNA) guidelines when performing construction in occupied buildings.

NOTES

1. Environmental Law Institute, *Building Healthy, High Performance Schools: A Review of Selected State and Local Initiatives*, 2003, http://www.elistore.org/reports_detail.asp?ID=10925
2. Patricia Lee, *Issue Brief: Summary and Analysis of State Policies on Asthma Education, Medications, and Triggers*, Center for Safe and Healthy Schools, National

Association of State Boards of Education, 2012, http://nasbe.org/project/center-for-safe-and-healthy-schools/ (accessed October 18, 2012).

3. American Society of Heating, Ventilating, and Air Conditioning Engineers, *ANSI/ASHRAE Standard 62.1-2010, Ventilation for Acceptable Indoor Air Quality*, 2010, http://www.ashrae.org/standards-research--technology/standards--guidelines (accessed October 18, 2012).
4. Maine Legislature, Title 5: Administrative Procedures and Services, c. 153, Pt. 4, §1742. Application of minimum air ventilation standards [1989, c. 502, Pt. A, §§15, 16 (AMD)] http://janus.state.me.us/legis/statutes/5/title5sec1742.html (accessed October 18, 2012).
5. Minnesota Statutes, Ch. 123B.71: Review and Comment for School District Construction, Subd 9.12. 2011, www.revisor.leg.state.mn.us/stats/123B/71.html (accessed October 18, 2012).
6. Workplace Safety and Health Program, Massachusetts Executive Office of Labor and Workforce Development, *Hazard Information Bulletin 392: Mechanical Ventilation Systems*, 2012, http://www.mass.gov/lwd/labor-standards/massachusetts-workplace-safety-and-health-program/hazard-info/392-mechanical-ventilation-systems-and-air.html (accessed October 18, 2012).
7. Workplace Safety and Health Program, Massachusetts Executive Office of Labor and *Workforce Development, Hazard* Information Bulletin 392: Mechanical Ventilation Systems, 2012, http://www.mass.gov/lwd/labor-standards/massachusetts-workplace-safety-and-health-program/hazard-info/392-mechanical-ventilation-systems-and-air.html
8. Workplace Safety and Health Program, Massachusetts Executive Office of Labor and Workforce Development, *Hazard Information Bulletin 389: Thermal Comfort Guidelines for Indoor Air*, 2012, http://www.mass.gov/lwd/labor-standards/massachusetts-workplace-safety-and-health-program/hazard-info/389-thermal-comfort-guidelines-for-indoor-air.html
9. California Department of Industrial Relations, Title 8 Ch. 4 Gr. 16 Article 107 §5142, Mechanically Driven Heating, Ventilating and Air Conditioning (HVAC) Systems to Provide Minimum Building Ventilation, 2012, http://www.dir.ca.gov/title8/5142.html (accessed October 18, 2012).
10. Risk Management Division, Minnesota Department of Administration, *Guidelines for Managing Indoor Air Quality*, http://www.admin.state.mn.us/risk/safety/documents/Minnesota_Guide_for_Managing_Indoor_Air_Quality.pdf (accessed October 18, 2012).
11. California Department of Industrial Relations, Title 8 Ch. 4 Gr. 16 Article 107 §5143, General Requirements of Mechanical Ventilation Systems, 2012, www.dir.ca.gov/title8/5143.html (accessed October 18, 2012).
12. American National Standards Institute (ANSI) and American Industrial Hygiene Association (AIHA), *American National Standard for Laboratory Ventilation Z9.5*, 2003. Available for purchase at www.ansi.org
13. American National Standards Institute (ANSI) and American Society for Heating, Refrigeration, and Air Conditioning Engineers, Inc. (ASHRAE), *ANSI/ASHRAE 110-1995: Method of Testing Performance of Laboratory Fume Hoods*. Available for purchase at www.ansi.org
14. American National Standards Institute (ANSI) and American Society for Heating, Refrigeration, and Air Conditioning Engineers, Inc. (ASHRAE), *ANSI/ASHRAE*

110-1995: Method of Testing Performance of Laboratory Fume Hoods, Section 5. Available for purchase at www.ansi.org

15. Vermont Department of Health, "Act 125: The Model Environmental Health Management Plan," http://healthvermont.gov/enviro/envision/plan.aspx (accessed October 18, 2012).
16. U.S. Environmental Protection Agency, "IAQ Design Tools for Schools," http://www.epa.gov/iaq/schooldesign (accessed October 18, 2012).
17. Connecticut General Statutes, Chapter 170, section 10-220, Subsection (a) (3), Duties of Boards of Education, http://search.cga.state.ct.us/surs/sur/htm/chap170.htm (accessed October 18, 2012).
18. Connecticut General Statutes, Chapter 170, Section 10-220, Subsection (a) (4), Duties of Boards of Education, http://search.cga.state.ct.us/surs/sur/htm/chap170.htm (accessed October 18, 2012).
19. Connecticut General Assembly, Substitute House Bill No. 6426, Public Act No. 03-220: An Act Concerning Air Quality in Schools, July 9, 2003, http://www.cga.ct.gov/2003/act/Pa/2003PA-00220-R00HB-06426-PA.htm (accessed October 18, 2012).
20. California Department of Industrial Relations, Title 8 Ch. 4, Sub Ch.7 Gr. 2 Article 9, *Sanitation*, http://www.dir.ca.gov/title8/sub7.html (accessed October 18, 2012).
21. General Assembly of the State of Vermont, H. 192 Act 125 Section 3(c)(2), Commissioners of Buildings and General Services, Education and Health, School Environmental Health Policy and Management Plan; Environmental Health Certificate, http://www.leg.state.vt.us/docs/2000/acts/act125.htm (accessed October 18, 2012).
22. U.S. Environmental Protection Agency, *Mold Remediation in Schools and Commercial Buildings* (EPA 402-K-01-001), September 2008, http://www.epa.gov/mold/mold_remediation.html (accessed October 18, 2012).
23. Massachusetts Multi-Agency Task Force on Schools, Massachusetts Health and Human Services, *The Massachusetts School Checklist*, February 2004, http://www.mass.gov/eohhs/docs/dph/environmental/iaq/schools-checklist.pdf (accessed October 18, 2012).
24. Workplace Safety and Health Program, Massachusetts Executive Office of Labor and Workforce Development, *Hazard Information Bulletin 416: Mold and Indoor Air Quality*, 2012, http://www.mass.gov/lwd/labor-standards/massachusetts-workplace-safety-and-health-program/hazard-info/416-mold-and-indoor-air-quality.html (accessed October 18, 2012).
25. General Assembly of the State of Vermont. Acts 0f 2000. No. 125. An Act Relating to Toxic Materials and Indoor Air Quality in Vermont Public Schools, 2000. http://www.leg.state.vt.us/docs/2000/acts/act125.htm accessed October 18, 2012.
26. Connecticut General Statutes, Chapter 170, Section 10-220(d), Duties of Boards of Education, http://search.cga.state.ct.us/surs/sur/htm/chap170.htm (accessed October 18, 2012).
27. State of Rhode Island and Providence Plantations Department of Elementary and Secondary Education and Department of Health, R16-21-SCHO: Rules and Regulations for School Health Programs, January 2009, http://sos.ri.gov/documents/archives/regdocs/released/pdf/DOH/5471.pdf (accessed October 12, 2012).

28. U.S. Environmental Protection Agency, "The Environmentally Preferable Purchasing Program," http://www.epa.gov/opptintr/epp/pubs/products/index.htm (accessed October 18, 2012).
29. Maine Department of Education and Department of Environmental Protection, *Hazardous Chemicals in Our Schools: Report to the Joint Standing Committee on Natural Resources*, January 2006, http://www.maine.gov/education/lres/scitech/safety.pdf (accessed October 18, 2012).
30. Green Seal, "Green Governments and Non-profits," http://www.greenseal.org/GreenGovernmentsAndNonProfits.aspx (accessed October 18, 2012).
31. National Councils for Occupational Safety and Health, "Local COSH Groups," http://www.coshnetwork.org/COSHGroupsList (accessed October 18, 2012).
32. U.S. Department of Labor, Occupational Safety and Health Administration, 29 CFR 1910.1200, Toxic and Hazardous Substances: Hazard Communication, http://www.osha.gov/pls/oshaweb/owadisp.show_document?p_table=standards&p_id=10099 (accessed October 18, 2012).
33. Massachusetts Executive Office of Labor and Workforce Development, Massachusetts Right to Know (RTK) Law, MGL 111F, http://www.mass.gov/lwd/labor-standards/occ-safety-and-health/right-to-know.html (accessed October 18, 2012).
34. U.S. Consumer Product Safety Commission, *An Update on Formaldehyde (Revision)*, 1997, http://www.cpsc.gov/cpscpub/pubs/725.pdf (accessed October 18, 2012).
35. Todd H. Dresser, U.S. Environmental Protection Agency, Region 7, "A Case Study of Environmental, Health & Safety Issues Involving the Burlington, MA Public School System," http://www.epa.gov/Region7/education_resources/teachers/ehsstudy/index.htm (accessed October 18, 2012).
36. Asthma Regional Council, "Building, Maintenance and Renovation," http://asthmaregionalcouncil.org/healthy-homes/move.html (accessed.October 18, 2012).
37. The Carpet and Rug Institute, "The Higher Standard for Indoor Air Quality," http://www.carpet-rug.org/commercial-customers/green-building-and-the-environment/green-label-plus/index.cfm (accessed October 18, 2012).
38. J. C. Chang, Z. Guo, R. Fortmann, and H. C. Lao, Characterization and Reduction of Formaldehyde Emissions from a Low-VOC Latex Paint, *Indoor Air, 12*(1), pp. 10-16, 2002.
39. California Department of Pesticide Regulation, "School Integrated Pest Management (IPM) Home Page," http://apps.cdpr.ca.gov/schoolipm/ (accessed October 18, 2012).
40. Massachusetts Department of Agricultural Resources (MDAR), "School IPM Program: Children's and Families Protection Act," www.mass.gov/agr/ipm (accessed October 18, 2012).
41. Green seal.
42. Massachusetts Executive Office for Administration and Finance, "Environmentally Preferable Products (EPP) Procurement Program," http://www.mass.gov/epp/products/cleaning.htm (accessed October 18, 2012).
43. Collaborative for High Performance Schools. Best Practices Manual, 2006. http://www.chps.net/dev/Drupal/node/288 (accessed October 18, 2012).
44. ANSI/Sheet Metal and Air Conditioning Contractors National Association, *IAQ Guidelines for Occupied Buildings under Construction* (2nd ed.), 2007, http://www.smacna.org/bookstore/index.cfm?fuseaction=search_results&cfid=9154107&cftoken=29570512 (accessed October 18, 2012).

45. U.S. EPA, "IAQ Design for Schools: Construction," http://www.epa.gov/iaq/school design/construction.html (accessed October 18, 2012).
46. Connecticut General Statutes, Chapter 170, Section 10-220, Subsection (d), Duties of Boards of Education, http://search.cga.state.ct.us/surs/sur/htm/chap170.htm (accessed October 18, 2012).
47. Maine Revised Statutes. Title 20, Part 3, Chapter 223, Subchapter 1, §6302, School Building Ventilation, http://janus.state.me.us/legis/statutes/20-A/title20-Asec6302.html (accessed October 18, 2012).
48. Maine Revised Statutes, Title 30-A, Part 2, Subpart 9, Chapter 225, Subchapter 3, §6006-F. School Revolving Renovation Fund, http://www.mainelegislature.org/legis/statutes/30-A/title30-Asec6006-F.html (accessed October 18, 2012).
49. Minnesota Planning: Environmental Quality Board, *Guide to Minnesota Environmental Review Rules*, 1998, http://www.mnplan.state.mn.us/pdf/rulguid3.pdf (accessed October 18, 2012).
50. American Society for Testing and Materials (ASTM), "E1527-05 Standard Practice for Environmental Site Assessments: Phase I Environmental Site Assessment Process," http://www.astm.org/Standards/E1527.htm (accessed October 18, 2012).
51. Maine Revised Statutes, RESOLVES: First Regular Session of the 120th, Chapter 50 H.P. 725-L.D. 945: Resolve, to Establish a Task Force to Examine the Establishment and Implementation of State Standards for Indoor Air Quality in Maine Schools, http://janus.state.me.us/legis/ros/lom/LOM120th/Res1-50/Res1-50-49.htm (accessed October 18, 2012).
52. Maine Revised Statutes, Title 20-A, Part7, Subpart 9, Chapter 609, §6006-F. §15912, Inspection of facility; compliance, http://janus.state.me.us/legis/statutes/20-A/title20-Asec15912.html (accessed October 18, 2012).
53. State of Rhode Island and Providence Plantations, Department of Elementary and Secondary Education and Department of Health, *R16-21-SCHO: Rules and Regulations for School Health Programs*, Part V, Section 42.1., January 2009, http://sos.ri.gov/documents/archives/regdocs/released/pdf/DOH/5471.pdf (accessed October 12, 2012).
54. State of Rhode Island and Providence Plantations, Department of Elementary and Secondary Education and Department of Health, *R16-21-SCHO: Rules and Regulations for School Health Programs*, Part V, Section 39.2., January 2009, http://sos.ri.gov/documents/archives/regdocs/released/pdf/DOH/5471.pdf (accessed October 12, 2012).

CHAPTER 13

Building the New Schoolhouse: The Massachusetts School Building Authority

Jennifer Ames and Charles Levenstein

In Chapter 1, Paulson and Barnett ask who is responsible for the environmental health of schools. The Massachusetts School Building Authority (MSBA), the product of liberals trying to bring organization and efficiency to school construction, is an "off-label" and only partial answer to the question. The MSBA, established in 2004, has lent its ear to health and safety advocates who saw an opportunity to implement regulations, guidelines, and education reforms at the level of school construction. The MSBA's progressiveness offers an intriguing example to localities and states across the United States facing the dual crisis of attacks on public education and financial inefficiency. However, the MSBA is still in its infancy and not without its critics among municipal auditors, architects, and building contractors. Time will tell whether the MSBA, viewed as a limited state pilot program, can survive and expand its integration of environmental health programs or whether the MSBA's initiative is only as good as its current leadership.

In August 2011 a report sponsored by the Twentieth Century Fund and the Economic Policy Institute described the enormity of the U.S. school building problem:

> The average U.S. public school building is 40 years old, and many are much older. The cost of maintaining nearly 100,000 public schools and facilities in good repair is enormous. According to the Government Accountability Office and the American Society of Civil Engineers, school districts have been under-spending on maintenance and repair for many years. Chronic deferred maintenance and repair can lead to energy inefficiencies, unsafe

> drinking water, water damage and moldy environments, poor air quality, inadequate fire alarms and fire safety, compromised building security, and structural dangers.
>
> By conservative estimates the accumulated backlog of deferred maintenance and repair amounts to at least $270 billion. Including the cost to "green-up" existing schools—and using less conservative assumptions—the cost of needed improvements to buildings and systems could exceed $500 billion [1].

Although most of the debate about school reform in the United States has focused on issues like high-stakes testing, vouchers, charter schools and the like, underlying the discussion is the substantial economic problem, including the deteriorating physical infrastructure of education. Large amounts of public monies are spent on construction of new schools and renovation of older ones, as well as on daily regular facilities maintenance. This is a big industry, and it is largely a creature of the public sector. As such, it is reasonable to expect that it has been greatly affected by the national and international resurgence of "neoliberalism," that is, the doctrines of conservative, market-oriented, anti-regulatory ideology and policy. It is also more than reasonable to ask the questions posed by Paulson and Barnett in Chapter 1 of this book: Who is responsible for the environmental health of children and staff in America's schools? They argue for federal and state initiatives to build "the capacity of the Environmental Protection Agency and the Centers for Disease Control and Prevention-designated and funded Pediatric Environmental Health Specialty Units (PEHSU) in responding to and evaluating risks to children's environmental health in schools" [2].

Beyond ideological considerations regarding public and private responsibility for schools, economic stagnation in the United States had consequences for public education.

> Total government spending on K-12 education as a percentage of GDP had risen in the 1960s and early 1970s, reaching 4.1 percent in 1975, only to fall to 3.6 percent a decade later, in 1985. The percentage of public school revenue coming from local government plummeted from 53 percent in 1965 to 44 percent in 1985 due to a widespread property tax revolt. . . . Schools, meanwhile, were forced to cope with growing deficits from the larger society. . . . Rising numbers of increasingly impoverished children arrived in the public schools, bringing with them more pressing needs, leading to greater strains on limited school resources [3].

Rather than alleviating the problem of school financing, privatization exacerbated the problem. Additionally, No Child Left Behind (NCLB) legislation passed in 2001 "put new burdens and expectations on schools and teachers, [but] total U.S. government spending on primary and secondary education as a percentage of GDP did not increase." The NCLB legislation, which required a controversial testing regime for students and an equally controversial system of school accountability, also "represented a massive, unfunded mandate, forcing district-run public schools to take on huge additional costs without the means to do so" [3]. While funding for K-12 education hardly increased at all, the demands of the legislation were such that a 20 to 35 percent increase would have been warranted. (For details of the law, see http://thomas.loc.gov/cgi-bin/bdquery/z?d107:HR0 0001:@@@D&Summ2=m&)

The neoliberal approaches to education, at least on paper, do not necessarily mean "starving the beast," as American conservatives have urged for the public sector generally. To the contrary, the "Washington Consensus," the broad set of recommendations shaping the practices of international financial institutions, urged that priorities in public expenditure be moved away "from subsidies and administration towards previously neglected fields with high economic returns," especially education [4]. Nevertheless, the actual practices have put great pressure on state and local budgets.

In the United States, the ineptness of public education bureaucracy, concerns about racial inequality in education expenditures, as well as alleged corruption in some states, fostered the search for reform. In 1988, New York City attempted to shed a history of alleged corruption and red tape by transferring school construction finance from the Department of Education to a new authority [5]. The New York School Construction Authority (NYSCA) was followed by similar restructuring and delegation of authority in other states, perhaps solving some of the inefficiencies of building schools but simultaneously casting school design even deeper into the outskirts of the curriculum- and performance-focused education debates. These new authorities and programs, sometimes completely independent from their states' departments of education, shook off bureaucratic burdens and political interests ostensibly to provide a reliable source of state funding for school construction and a commitment to efficiency and accountability in the process.

On its face, the Massachusetts School Building Authority (MSBA) had all the trappings of an agency bent on bringing business-like efficiency to school building finance, just like its NYSCA predecessor. However, the MSBA's mission did not end at making schools affordable but also "safe, sound, and sustainable learning environments." As such, it reached beyond the fiscal expertise of its staff to include health and safety advocates in creating regulations and guidelines for new school buildings. With participation by school districts, the MSBA has ushered in a technocratic process of school construction conditional only on the assessments of the impact the physical condition of a school has on its occupants. Thus, primarily created in response to bureaucratic and fiscal crisis, the MSBA has moved into areas of environmental health and education reform, elevating the relevance of school design in education policy and offering an intriguing example of the opportunities approachable at the level of school construction.

ORIGINS OF THE MASSACHUSETTS SCHOOL BUILDING AUTHORITY

The circumstances leading to the MSBA's creation are similar to those of the larger school building crisis that affects all states. As reported in *The Boston Globe*, the story of Massachusetts's school building finance was one of chronic problems for the state's budget. By 2004, school building projects in the Commonwealth were at a standstill [6]. The Department of Education (DoE) had nearly 400 projects pending on its school building assistance program. The section of the DoE responsible for this program was administered by three staff who could not keep up with a surge of construction projects in the 1990s and as a result, the funding system allegedly became lax and unreliable [7, 8]. For school districts hoping to start a building project or modernize an existing school, the wait time for state funds could be as long as 10 to 15 years while the DoE slowly dealt with a $4 billion backlog. At this rate, existing schools would continue to deteriorate under the weight of larger class sizes and aging energy systems. While school building finance had been under the DoE's purview since the 1940s, the unwieldy waitlist was drawing criticism. When, in 2003, the DoE placed a moratorium on new building projects, the Commissioner of Education Paul Driscoll justified the move: "We've really reached a crisis stage" [9].

Despite attempts to fix the system under Governor Celluci in 2000, the system limped along another four years before Governor Mitt Romney (2003-2007) announced that education was one of his top priorities. This political climate was in part shaped by the attention around *Hancock v. Driscoll*, a case brought by Julie Hancock, a public school student in Brockton, Massachusetts, against the Commissioner of Education in 1999 for not equitably distributing funds to the poorest schools in the Commonwealth. The 2004 ruling by the Suffolk Superior Court of Massachusetts, in favor of the complaining school districts, found that the state was not upholding its constitutional duty to provide the resources needed for an adequate public education [10, 11]. The verdict identified overcrowding as one of the major obstacles to education, and consequently spurred the Massachusetts state legislature to get the school building program back on track. Though the Supreme Judicial Court of Massachusetts later overturned the decision in February of 2005, neither the state nor the overwhelmed staff at DoE questioned the call for reform.

However, deciding the design of the reform was not without disagreement between the legislature controlled by Democrats and the Republican governor. Reform discussions began when Romney put forth a plan in January 2004. He proposed borrowing money for school projects over a 40-year term instead of the then-current 20 years, which he expected would save the state $150 million in 2004 and allow every project on the waitlist to be paid off by 2009 [12]. However, State Treasurer and future gubernatorial candidate Tim Cahill, working on a plan of his own, anticipated Romney's financing plan would merely shift the tax burden to future generations and raise the overall cost to taxpayers.

Cahill's alternative, unveiled a few months later, proposed a more drastic overhaul of the current system, borrowing to pay off the waitlist in 3.5 years and dedicating sales tax revenue to sustain future projects.

In April 2004, the Democrats in the Massachusetts legislature introduced a bill that adopted Cahill's proposals. In an election year, as one reporter noted, "Both the Democrats and Romney recognize[d] the political resonance of a need that affects nearly every city and town in Massachusetts" [13]. Romney signed the Cahill bill into law that summer, establishing the Massachusetts School Building Authority [14]. Cahill served as the first MSBA chairman in 2004.

The MSBA's main directive was to reform the funding process for school building projects. It began by gradually shifting 20 percent of the state's sales tax revenue to a school building fund. Previously, the DoE's school building assistance program collected funds from overall state revenues, which can be less stable and do not grow 4 to 6 percent a year the way sales tax revenues typically did at that time [15]. A board of seven members representing the state's education, design, and finance leaders was appointed to steer the Authority. Also among the board members were designees of the Department of Education and the Secretary of Administration and Finance. The MSBA worked closely with the staff at the Department of Education, tapping their years of experience administering the former school building program. In addition to the Board, an executive director appointed by the Board's chairperson would manage a staff tasked with overseeing the MSBA's administrative needs and general operations. The Director would work closely with the Board to ensure the smooth implementation of the latter's policies and directives.

The financial fulcrum of the legislation rests on the transfer of power from the DoE to the state treasurer who serves as the chair of the MSBA; moving school building finances to the Treasury office, which already managed other state public debt related to road and building projects at the time the MSBA was established, seemed like a logical consolidation of authority. The MSBA inherited 427 building projects with an estimated cost of $4.2 billion. The agency was required to handle "the largest capital grant program operated by the commonwealth" and increased its staff from three to over 70, as well as marshalling other resources required for the task [16]. Primary among the Cahill law's purposes was:

> . . . to create an authority to achieve the objectives of effective management and planning of the commonwealth's investments in school building assets, promoting positive educational outcomes, ensuring the health, safety, security and well-being of students, easing and preventing overcrowding, maintaining good repair, efficient and economical construction and maintenance, financial sustainability of the school building assistance program, thoughtful community development, smart growth and accessibility [16].

Its first director, Katherine Craven, recruited from her position as Director of Policy for the Massachusetts House of Representatives, was instrumental in implementing these objectives. As one business writer described her task, "MSBA was the proverbial bull-in-the-china-shop from the get-go" [17]. In conjunction with the board of directors, the new staff of the MSBA swiftly approached cleanup of the state's school construction mess with what was described as "business-like" rigor.

Counting schools with completed or already launched projects, the waitlist for reimbursement included about 1,200 projects worth at least $9.2 billion. The first task was to place a moratorium on all building project applications until 2007 while the MSBA chipped away at the projects already in the pipeline. The second task was to conduct a comprehensive audit of more than 600 projects to monitor costs and prevent overpayments, a problem the Department of Education encountered because it lacked the staff and resources to audit budgets and inspect construction sites efficiently. The MSBA ordered the audits in preparation for the state Treasury to sell bonds to raise money [18]. Meanwhile sales tax revenue went towards paying off the debt.

The Cahill Bill that enabled the MSBA also specified the establishment of a School Building Advisory Board to provide additional guidance from non-governmental agencies. The prescribed make-up of the Board includes the State Auditor and Inspector General or their designees, and members from 15 organizations representing educators, superintendents, architects, and contractors, among other vested interests. The director of the MSBA serves as the Secretary. The intended purpose of the Advisory Board is to:

> . . . assist the authority in the development of general policy regarding school building construction, renovation, reconstruction, maintenance and facility space, preservation of open space and minimization of loss of open space, thoughtful community development, cost management and [to] provide technical advice and input to the authority. The advisory board shall meet at least quarterly [19].

As of the summer of 2012, one member of the Advisory Board informed the authors that the group had not convened in the three years since his appointment. According to this informant, the Board serves a minimal role and has neither been invited to nor apparently intends to make a concerted effort to contribute to the MSBA's decision-making. Without direction or communication from the MSBA, the Board has had no focus on which to mobilize its efforts. At best, Advisory Board members independently report back to the MSBA from their community experiences, but do not collaborate with other Board members to inform and shape MSBA policy.

THE BULL IN THE CHINA SHOP

The first years of the MSBA were focused on building what was already promised, but the Authority had the equally important task of deciding how schools would be built from that point onward. The MSBA intended to function not only as a dispenser of funds but also as a "bully pulpit" for the promotion of a wide range of good practices in school construction. In addition, one of Craven's goals was to make the process transparent, and hence the MSBA launched an online database where citizens could monitor project costs. A variety of stakeholders including representatives of teachers' unions and the Massachusetts Healthy Schools Network were invited to help shape the regulations for the new agency. The statute which created the MSBA placed great emphasis on planning, due diligence, and the prioritization of scarce MSBA resources for the school building projects that demonstrated the most need. To assess these needs, three main areas emerged as central to MSBA's decision-making:

1. The Needs Survey by the MSBA identified trouble spots in school districts. A team of design and engineering professionals visited each school eligible for MSBA funding to evaluate several key factors including building systems conditions, general physical environment, and space utilization. The Needs Survey results were to be an important look at the current condition of school facilities, identifying needs that might meet the statutory priorities for funding.
2. A Statement of Interest (SOI) submitted by the school district indicated its construction needs. While the Needs Survey identified trouble spots in the state's schools, the school district had sole discretion to initiate a building project by submitting a statement of interest to the MSBA. The SOI format allowed school districts to describe current and foreseeable facility inadequacies but emphasized a checklist of the MSBA's major priorities, notably serious structural problems and present or imminent overcrowding (see Table 1). The MSBA did not limit the number of SOIs that a district could submit, except that the district could submit only one per school building in any filing period. Each district was required to designate one SOI as its "district priority SOI" for consideration and due diligence efforts by the MSBA. An SOI in the MSBA capital pipeline was presumed to be the district's priority until the time of project completion. In order to show community support for the submission of an SOI, the MSBA required endorsement by the local school committee and, except in the case of a regional school district, the responsible municipal body (e.g., City Council, Aldermen, or Board of Selectmen) authorizing the Superintendent of Schools to submit an SOI to the MSBA [20].
3. Upon receipt of the SOI, the MSBA investigated the conditions and needs of the school district. These assessments, more focused and comprehensive than the broad-sweeping Needs Survey, typically included a review of the SOI and any supporting documents, a review of historical and projected enrollment trends, a review of educational programs, and/or site visits to the school facility performed by a team of staff, architects, and engineers

Table 1. Statement of Interest Priorities
(Superintendent to Indicate Which Apply)

1. Replacement or renovation of a building which is structurally unsound or otherwise in a condition seriously jeopardizing the health and safety of school children, where no alternative exists.
2. Elimination of existing severe overcrowding.
3. Prevention of the loss of accreditation.
4. Prevention of severe overcrowding expected to result from increased enrollments.
5. Replacement, renovation, or modernization of school facility systems, such as roofs, windows, boilers, heating and ventilation systems, to increase energy conservation and decrease energy related costs in a school facility.
6. Short term enrollment growth.
7. Replacement of or addition to obsolete buildings in order to provide for a full range of programs consistent with state and approved local requirements.
8. Transition from court-ordered and approved racial balance school districts to "walk-to"or other school districts.

Source: Massachusetts School Building Authority, *Statement of Interest System: User Guide for School District Users for Fiscal Year 2012,* accessed at http://www.massschoolbuildings.org/sites/default/files/edit-contentfile/Guidelines_Forms/Guidelines_Policies/2012%20Statement%20of%20Interest%20User%20Guide.pdf

with experience in school facilities and educational curricula. With the information gathered, the MSBA Board then voted on which projects to invite into the eligibility phase, which is a series of steps that eventually leads to funding.

All three of these factors stress issues of structural/mechanical soundness of the school and overcrowding. For school districts, these crises took prominence over less visible environmental hazards such as mold or poor indoor air quality. Though environmental health concerns were not the main priority of school districts, the MSBA indirectly addressed these issues in schools by writing them into the regulations for new buildings. Furthermore, the MSBA would later introduce auxiliary building incentives and programs that emphasized environmental repairs in schools where overcrowding and roof collapse were not overriding issues. The checklist of the SOI, capturing these visible issues, aimed to rectify the legacy of "lousy construction" and negligent building maintenance that had grown under the DoE [21].

MSBA IN OPERATION

The rigor of the Authority's systematic selection of schools was made possible by its position outside the bureaucratic and political complications that had sunk the DoE. Accountable to no one but its own staff and directorship, and equipped with stable revenue from the state sales tax, the MSBA had created a series of steps and criteria to streamline and bring transparency to the construction of public schools. Furthermore, with support from the State Treasurer, the education reformers saw an opportunity to implement building standards and push an educational agenda, at least to the extent that it interfaced with new construction and/or major renovation of school facilities. School districts, galvanized by the restoration of state funding for school construction, were willing to play by the MSBA's rules so long as the price remained within what they considered affordable bounds.

While the MSBA put forth certain requirements pertaining to air quality, enrollment-appropriate square footage, and airtight construction, among others, the school district could participate in the selection of its project team. The eligibility phase for a school district invited into the capital pipeline begins with a feasibility study. The district is tasked with creating a building committee of community members and selecting an owner's project manager (OPM) and architect who also meet the MSBA's approval. With the help of its designer, the school district performs a feasibility study to propose a renovation or new construction project to address the issues laid out in the SOI. Vetting the members of the project team and centralizing coordination on the OPM were measures adopted to avoid the disorganization and corruption that were alleged to have colored the DoE's system of subcontracting and oversight.

At all steps of the planning and building process, a school district, its designer, and its construction team are answerable to the MSBA and the latter's discretionary funding. Even though the MSBA reimburses at considerably lower rates than the State had previously, the funds are a necessity to the majority of communities; few if any school districts have budgets that could bear shouldering the full cost of a school construction project. Given this great financial dependence, the MSBA technical staff had relatively free rein to set the terms of school construction. The staff began by drafting guidelines for health and safety issues such as indoor air quality, square footage, and proper siting. At the urging of advocates who recognized the value of this opportunity, the guidelines turned into requirements for all new buildings intended to receive MSBA funding [21]. Katherine Craven, the MSBA director, "was ready to listen" to progressive organizations such as the Massachusetts Teachers Association, the Healthy Schools Coalition, the Massachusetts Coalition for Occupational Safety and Health (MassCOSH), and the Parent-Teacher Association (PTA). Flying under the political radar, the MSBA advanced environmental health from what some considered a financial bully pulpit [22]. This would further develop, with the introduction of the Science Lab initiative and Green Repair program, to define the MSBA's stick-and-carrot approach to other educational reforms affecting not only health and safety, but curriculum agendas and professional development as well [22].

The period in which the MSBA began drafting its building requirements and reimbursement policies coincided with new developments in the field of school design. "Green," energy-efficient technologies were becoming more attractive and affordable and the LEED rating system was coming into vogue. The Leadership in Energy and Environmental Design (LEED) system, developed by the U.S. Green Building Council in 2000, provides guidance for construction of high-performing buildings in terms of environmental impact and energy efficiency. The LEED guidelines address issues such as classroom acoustics, air quality, mold prevention, and environmental site assessment [23]. "The confluence of these movements," as Phil Katz, a member of the MSBA Advisory Committee and former head of the Brookline Teachers' Association, as well as consultant to the major teachers' unions in Massachusetts, describes, "was happening naturally" [24]. In 2008, as the backlog dwindled, the Authority's focus shifted to promoting this "greener" environmentally friendly and energy-efficient school construction, a movement whose popularity predated the MSBA. In fact, several pro-active school districts, opposed to languishing under the DoE's reimbursement process, had taken advantage of competitive grants from the Massachusetts Technology Collaborative, which awarded up to $650,000 toward the design, planning, and construction of schools using renewable energy sources. The MSBA added new vigor to this initiative in 2009 by introducing a reimbursement point system to increase the appeal of designs that incorporated criteria published by the Massachusetts Collaborative for High Performance Schools (MA-CHPS). The criteria pertain to aspects of school environmental health such as design elements that promote air quality, environmentally friendly building materials, and ample natural light, among others. They also began a pilot "model schools" program and added a reimbursement incentive to schools that chose to adapt a school design prototype rather than draw up their building project from scratch. Model schools increased the affordability of construction by streamlining the process.

Uncommon and underfunded by the DoE, renovation projects rebounded under the MSBA. This was in part facilitated by the MSBA staff's assistance to schools in handling feasibility studies, thorough budget auditing, and careful planning. Renovations further thrived following introduction of the Green Repair program. The Green Repair program, touting the cost savings of installing or repairing energy-efficient heating systems or insulating windows, offered a cheaper way to improve schools without the expense of a complete rebuild. Under the DoE, the culture of allowing schools to deteriorate to the point of disrepair meant funded projects were almost exclusively new buildings.

However, the MSBA, with its meticulous audits, Needs Survey, and insistence on each school having building maintenance plans, made repairs a more appealing and feasible option for school districts. The Green Repair program and a new Science Lab initiative targeted and facilitated the growth of renovation proposals.

The primary focus of the Science Lab initiative was to boost science education in Massachusetts. As the current State Treasurer Steven Grossman remarks, "ensuring that our high school students have access to a top-notch, 21st century science curriculum and facilities not only better prepares our kids for the demands of an evolving job market, but it will also enhance the future competitiveness of the Commonwealth" [25]. However, as Terry Kwan, MSBA board member and one of the driving architects of the initiative, explained to the authors, the call to revamp science education coincided with her and her colleagues' efforts at the National Science Teacher Association to update school lab safety guidelines. Rolling these guidelines into the Science Lab initiative helped mobilize the stakeholders on the task force and gave context to promoting safety as a top priority of all the design requirements and "best practices." The Science Lab Task Force, which included MSBA Board members and staff, Department of Elementary and Secondary Education staff, science educators, science and technology consultants, science lab safety consultants, local architects, and construction management consultants, contributed to the development of "science lab prototypes that are curriculum-driven, accommodate all science disciplines through flexibility, and provide a safe learning environment for students" [25]. Health and safety concerns in the guidelines addressed the implementation of appropriate square footage to prevent lab accidents, adoption of green chemistry, proper ventilation, and safe storage and positioning of lab equipment and materials within the lab space and adjacent facilities. In addition to these safety design elements, schools also have to provide curriculum plans to demonstrate the new lab's enrichment of students' experiences and teachers' professional development. While a voluntary program still in its infancy, the Science Lab initiative continues to be a selective and competitive application process with only 10 schools invited into the capital pipeline as of June 2012 [26].

New construction needs, even repairs, had to conform to tougher standards and were always considered in a holistic view of the school district. The MSBA would not approve a district's proposal of a science lab renovation, for instance, if the whole school was in such bad shape that it would need replacement in a few years. Likewise, the MSBA could require a school to install a new ventilation system along with a science lab renovation or submission of curriculum or professional development plans from science teachers [22]. Such exacting management was necessary for an agency averse to financial waste and committed to optimized school buildings. The MSBA's regulations and guidelines pertaining to environmental health are summarized in Table 2.

Table 2. MSBA Environmental Guidelines and Regulations

Indoor Air Quality Guidelines (adopted 2006)

- Protection of building materials
- Limits on vehicle idling

Best Practices for Maintenance

- Resources: EPA Tools for Schools
- Resources: NCES School Maintenance Guide
- Other resources re: energy saving

Green Design (Sustainable Schools) Guidelines

- Mass CHPS Guidelines
- LEED System for Schools Guidelines

Science Lab Guidelines (2001)

Source: Massachusetts School Building Authority, "Guidelines, Policies, & Perquisite Forms," http://www.massschoolbuildings.org/guidelines (accessed October 9, 2012).

DISCUSSION

The very effective national attack on public sector budgets by conservative political forces (the "neoliberals") exerted great pressure on the nation's school systems. In 2006, the Texas legislature was reconsidering the way in which the state distributed school construction monies and collected data on the variety of arrangements across the country [27].

Only four states refrained from providing support to localities in funding school construction: Nebraska, Nevada, Oklahoma, and South Dakota. Across those states that did provide some form of support, there was a range of revenue sources, types of aid, and systems for oversight. Environmental concerns, as far as we could tell from the Texas review, were not the top priority in any of the states. Overcrowding, race discrimination and, at least in one case, alleged gangster involvement, provided the rationales for the arrangements. Thus there is really no state model aimed primarily at dealing with the "toxic schoolhouse." In fact, the MSBA was intended to solve quite a different set of problems—although, once the new agency was created, it provided an off-label vehicle for environmental reform as well as a remedy for bureaucratic inefficiency.

A teacher's union representative who has served on the MSBA Advisory Board commented: "The MSBA is less bureaucratic in a way that is more efficient and less political than the DoE. They don't have to deal with the commissioner of education. . . . [The leadership] are technocrats . . . more like a business. . . . Things move a lot more smoothly, school districts get a lot more help." He noted, however, that the Advisory Board ". . . is not consulted though, so in a way, stakeholders are not included as much as they should be." The Advisory Board had not met for the preceding three years.

While it is still early to evaluate the successes and/or failures of the MSBA, our interviews with representatives of advocacy groups, teachers' union representatives, and a board member, as well as documentary review, have found few complaints about the MSBA. All agree that the MSBA has had an open ear to reforming building requirements. Apparently the construction unions, however, were not at all involved in MSBA discussions, so construction safety, for instance, is not in the MSBA regulations. We were told that there was criticism from municipal auditors, architects, and contractors, and it was evident that there had been a shift of power away from the previous bureaucratic regime—and from the insider political game. The requirement that localities have their own technical assistance—a project manager who meets MSBA standards—is a strong support for democratic involvement in technical decision-making. Perhaps what is most striking is that the reform that MSBA represents is not consistent with the market-oriented neoliberal agenda that has encroached upon public policy since the Reagan Administration. The MSBA appears to be the brainchild of liberal technocrats who were given a loose rein under Romney's term as governor of Massachusetts [28].

CRITIQUE AND THE WAY FORWARD

As of July 2012, the MSBA had completed final audits on 847 projects representing a total of $15 billion in submitted costs since its inception in 2004. With 305 schools in the capital pipeline and another 280 SOIs representing 121 school districts on the review table, the MSBA continues to function to capacity, fulfilling a critical need in the Commonwealth [26]. Of the 90 projects to be completed in 2012, 68 were green repairs. Furthermore, 40 percent of the SOIs currently under review are resubmittals compared to 26 percent first-time submissions. At the end of a construction project, the MSBA also funds at 100 percent the commissioning of an independent third party to test the buildings systems, structural integrity, and overall operation to confirm quality assurance. School districts submit maintenance plans to carry on the effort after that.

The MSBA's model of careful planning, appropriate construction, and incentivized building programs has transformed and invigorated school construction in Massachusetts. In order to work so efficiently and with such progressive development, the MSBA necessarily needed to be excised from the Department of Education; the politicized environment of the latter would have precluded such a steady stream of funding and auditing. Money from a direct source of tax revenue gave the MSBA leadership room to operate outside of narrow political constraints as well as private economic interests. Reforming the finance system could have been the end goal, and the MSBA could have run its streamlined course in perpetuity. However, it took a more progressive and thoughtful course made possible by leadership willing to listen to health and safety advocates. Katherine Craven, the first director, has been widely credited with steering the MSBA in this direction, and the current Board of Directors, whose membership has not changed much since 2004, has carried this spirit forward. However, the MSBA is only as progressive as its leadership and has no inherent mandate to develop its environmental health agenda. For example, the green repair program's popularity is primarily incentivized by the cost savings of lower energy bills rather than by advocacy for environmental conservation. While these repairs often improve the environmental health of the school through improved air quality or by removing old caulking laced with PCBs, these health benefits come via an indirect solution. Historical and palpable issues such as overcrowding and structural unsoundness invite straightforward fixes, but the "invisible hazards" of a school building are just as detrimental to students and employees yet are not actively targeted. Perhaps one area worthy of investigation is whether the model school program disproportionately lowers costs to communities without environmental obstacles, where site remediation is not a commonplace complication. Can the MSBA's mission to improve accessibility to safe and structurally sound schools be better tailored to environmental justice districts where environmental problems might require more expensive solutions? The MSBA arguably has the bureaucratic and legislative freedom to address the issues of the toxic schoolhouse head-on but is heavily dependent on the personality and commitments of its leadership.

At the same time, the MSBA's exercise of its financial power, a bully pulpit, and stick-and-carrot approach to enforcing better school construction, does open it up to questions of accountability. As a quasi-independent agency under the Treasurer with limited input from the DoE, at what point could the MSBA's secondary agenda be seen as encroaching on democratic prerogatives—or an abuse of legislative activism? After just eight years, the MSBA has rescued Massachusetts's school construction business and galvanized enthusiasm and confidence in its funding program. While it may be too early to evaluate completed projects for adequacy and sustainability, the success of the programs is promising. The MSBA's off-label efforts to improve school physical environments beyond just making them big enough and able to stand, may provide a translatable model for harnessing school construction regulations to introduce health and safety measures. While conditions in Massachusetts were ripe for these activities to develop naturally, the MSBA's policies are adaptable to other independent building authorities and highlight the benefits of taking school building construction outside the ring of politicized funding.

Nevertheless, the MSBA could deal only with new projects, not with the deplorable condition of the state's school facilities as a whole. Further, the rules that seemed to deal with school districts in an even-handed way mask the imbalance in resources and needs between the old industrial cities and the newer suburban communities. Only one "priority" project per district is permitted even if the problems are much more widespread in the particular community. In addition, MSBA does not address the less dramatic (or visible) situations where major renovation is not required but which threaten the health and welfare of students and staff. MSBA has no role in enforcement of AHERA (asbestos management requirements under the Asbestos Hazard Emergency Response Act) integrated pest management, green cleaners, and so forth. Thus, MSBA is a useful step—but it does not meet the continuing need for audit and oversight of environmental conditions in Massachusetts schools. Apparently there is still no one in the schools in charge of environmental health of children (and staff); that is the answer to the question posed by Paulson and Barnett at the outset of this book and this chapter.

NOTES

1. Mary Filardo, Jared Bernstein, and Ross Eisenbrey, *Creating Jobs Through FAST!, A Proposed New Infrastructure Program to Repair America's Public Schools*," Twentieth Century Fund and the Economic Policy Institute, August 11, 2011.
2. J. Paulson and C. Barnett, "Who's in Charge of Children's Environmental Health at School?" *New Solutions: A Journal of Environmental and Occupational Health Policy* 20(1), 2010.
3. John Bellamy Foster, "Education and the Structural Crisis of Capital: The U.S. Case," *Monthly Review*, July 1, 2011.
4. World Health Organization, "Washington Consensus," http://www.who.int/trade/glossary/story094/en/index.html (accessed May 31, 2012).
5. Selwyn Raab, "School-Building Agency Changes the Old Rules," *The New York Times*, October 8, 1989, http://www.nytimes.com/1989/10/18/nyregion/school-building-agency-changes-the-old-rules.html (accessed July 9, 2012).
6. Franco Ordonez, "State Moratorium Puts School Projects in Doubt, Door Shut on Reimbursement Program," *The Boston Globe*, February 23, 2003.
7. Robert Preer, "Rush to Build Schools Puts Strain on State Funds," *The Boston Globe*, January 2, 2000.
8. Beth Daley, "New Schools Test Towns: Replacing Old Facilities is Expensive and Complicated—and Lack of State Oversight Often Results in Shoddy Construction and Huge Overruns," *The Boston Globe*, June 25, 2000.
9. Anand Vaishnav and Megan Tench, "Program on School Aid Takes Timeout," *The Boston Globe*, February 12, 2003.
10. Margot Botsford, "*Hancock v. Driscoll:* Final Conclusions and Recommendations," Massachusetts Supreme Judicial Court, April 26, 2004.
11. Brenda J. Buote, "Education Officials Hope Ruling Spurs Action," *The Boston Globe*, May 6, 2004.
12. Scott S. Greenberger, "Romney Offers Plan to Rebuild Schools," *The Boston Globe*, January 17, 2004.

13. Scott S. Greenberger, "Plan Eyed to Fund Work on Schools," *The Boston Globe*, April 11, 2004.
14. Alexander Reid, "School Building Fund Replenished; Overhaul to Speed Reimbursements," *The Boston Globe*, August 12, 2004.
15. Peter DeMarco, "New School-Building Law Adds More Certainty," *The Boston Globe*, July 29, 2004.
16. 188th General Court of the Commonwealth of Massachusetts, "General Laws/ Section 1," http://www.malegislature.gov/Laws/GeneralLaws/PartI/TitleXII/Chapter 70B/Section1 (accessed June 19, 2012).
17. Craig M. Douglas, "Massachusetts School Building Authority Chief Puts Reins on Spending," *Boston Business Journal*, June 3, 2011, http://www.bizjournals.com/ boston/print-edition/2011/06/03/massachusetts-school-building.html (accessed July 6, 2012).
18. Maria Sacchetti, "State Plans School Construction Probe," *The Boston Globe,* March 31, 2005.
19. Statutes Relating to the Massachusetts School Building Authority, Chapter 70B, Section 3(a), 187th General Court of the Commonwealth of Massachusetts, http:// www.massschoolbuildings.org/sites/default/files/edit-contentfile/Guidelines_Forms/ Statutes_Regulations/MSBA%20Enabling%20Legislation%20POSTED%2011%2022 %2010.pdf (accessed September 19, 2012).
20. Massachusetts School Building Authority, "Statements of Interest," http://www.mass schoolbuildings.org/building/prerequisites/SOI_overview (accessed October 9, 2012).
21. Sarah Gibson (attorney who works closely with the Teachers' Union), personal communication, June 21, 2012.
22. Terry Kwan (MSBA Board of Directors), personal communication, June 29, 2012.
23. U.S. Green Building Council, *LEED 2009 for Schools New Constructions and Major Renovations*, 2008, http://www.usgbc.org/ShowFile.aspx?DocumentID=8872 (accessed October 9, 2012).
24. Phil Katz (MSBA Advisory Committee Member), personal communication, June 18, 2012.
25. State Treasurer Steven Grossman, as quoted in Massachusetts State Building Authority, "MSBA Announces $60M High School Science Lab Initiative," September 28, 2011, http://www.massschoolbuildings.org/news_events/9.28.11Board/Science_ labs (accessed October 9, 2012).
26. Massachusetts School Building Authority, "Presentation to MA Association of Superintendents," July 12, 2012, http://www.massschoolbuildings.org/sites/default/files/ edit-contentfile/Public%20Presentations/MASS_7_12_12_FINAL_no_web_cover. pdf (accessed October 9, 2012).
27. Texas Legislative Council, *Facts at a Glance: State Roles in Financing Public School Facilities*, December 2006, http://www.tlc.state.tx.us/pubspol/OnlineFinancePub Sch.pdf (accessed October 9, 2012).
28. Anonymous informant familiar with Massachusetts Division of Capital Asset Management, personal communication, July 10, 2012.

Contributors

JENNIFER AMES is a graduate student and research assistant in the Department of Environmental Health at the Boston University School of Public Health.

CLAIRE BARNETT is the founding Executive Director of Healthy Schools Network, Inc. (HSN), a national environmental health not-for-profit research, education, and advocacy organization, and the Coordinator of the national Coalition for Healthier Schools. Convening partners into a national Coalition, she shaped and won enactment of the federal Healthy and High Performance Schools Act in 2002, which codified school design criteria and established a National Priority Study on the impacts of decayed facilities on children. She also led the campaign for the federal High Performance Green Buildings Act of 2007 that advances children's environmental health at school. She has chaired two EPA work groups and led briefings for Congress and the White House. In 2005, HSN received awards for its informational clearinghouse and for promoting Indoor Air Quality in schools.

PHIL BROWN, PhD is University Distinguished Professor of Sociology and Health Sciences at Northeastern university, where he directs the Social Science Environmental Health Research Institute. He is the author of *No Safe Place: Toxic Waste, Leukemia, and Community Action* and *Toxic Exposures: Contested Illnesses and the Environmental Health Movement* and coeditor of *Illness and the Environment: A Reader in Contested Medicine, Social Movements in Health* and *Contested Illnesses: Citizens, Science, and Health Social Movements.* His current research includes biomonitoring and household exposure, social policy concerning flame retardants, ethics of reporting research data to participants, and health social movements.

MARLENE CAMACHO served as an intern with the Boston Urban Asthma Coalition.

ALISON COHEN, a 2009-2010 Fulbright scholar to the European Union and 2008 Udall Scholar for environmental leadership, graduated magna cum laude, with honors, from Brown University in Community Health and Education Policy; she was affiliated with the Brown University Superfund Research Program's Community Outreach Core. She holds an MPH in epidemiology and biostatistics from University of California Berkeley, and is a doctoral student in epidemiology at UC Berkeley.

MARC EDWARDS, PhD, is the Charles Lunsford Professor of Civil Engineering at Virginia Tech, where he teaches environmental engineering and applied aquatic chemistry. In 2004, *Time* magazine dubbed him "The Plumbing Professor" and listed him among the world's four most important "innovators" in water. He was awarded the White House Presidential Faculty Fellowship in 1996 and a MacArthur Fellowship in 2007. He was president of the Association of Environmental and Engineering Science Professors and has testified to the U.S. Congress about lead in Washington D.C.'s drinking water. His research group currently focuses on internal corrosion processes in home plumbing, which costs U.S. consumers billions of dollars a year and jeopardizes the safety of drinking water.

KYLE ESDAILLE is a doctoral student in the Morgan State University School of Community Health and Policy's Public Health Program with a primary interest and focus in environmental health.

SARAH GIBSON is an attorney who for more than 15 years has represented and trained unions, individual employees, and employers on the technical and legal dimensions of health and safety issues, including indoor air quality, asbestos, toxic exposures, workplace accommodations for employees, work-related disability retirement, handicap discrimination, and collective bargaining/contract issues. Ms. Gibson has an MS degree from the Department of Work Environment at the University of Massachusetts Lowell (1994) and is a graduate of Northeastern University School of Law (1982) and Wellesley College (1976). Before starting her own practice, Ms. Gibson was a staff attorney with the Massachusetts Teachers Association (MTA). She is co-chair of the Boston Society of Architects' Indoor Air Quality Committee, is a consultant to the MTA's Environmental Health & Safety Committee, and serves on the Massachusetts Healthy Schools Network.

TOLLE GRAHAM is an organizer and the Healthy Schools Coordinator for the Massachusetts Coalition for Occupational Safety and Health (MassCOSH). She is a member of the United Steelworkers Local 9358-1.

ROBERT F. HERRICK has a BA degree in Chemistry from the College of Wooster, an MS in Environmental Health Science from the University of Michigan, and an SD in Industrial Hygiene from the Harvard School of Public Health. He is certified in the comprehensive practice of industrial hygiene and is a Fellow of the American Industrial Hygiene Association. Dr. Herrick is past chair of the American Conference of Governmental Industrial Hygienists, and past president of the International Occupational Hygiene Association. Before joining the faculty at the Harvard School of Public Health, Dr. Herrick spent 17 years at the National Institute for Occupational Safety and Health (NIOSH) where he conducted occupational health research, specializing in exposure assessment for epidemiologic studies. He was the NIOSH liaison to the U.S. Environmental

Protection Agency Science Advisory Board, Indoor Air Quality and Total Human Exposure Committee. He has participated in several expert committees and review panels, most recently in the National Academy of Sciences Committee to Review the Health Effects in Vietnam Veterans of Exposure to Herbicides.

YANNA LAMBRINIDOU, PhD, is president of Parents for Nontoxic Alternatives, a local children's environmental health organization in Washington, D.C. As a medical ethnographer, her research interests lie at the intersection of culture, the politics of knowledge, and environmental health and justice. She has worked on contested areas in matters of illness and medicine, with a focus on negotiation processes between affected communities and institutions responsible for their health. She has studied end-of-life care; alternative and complementary medicine in the treatment of childhood cancer; and lead-contaminated drinking water, a source of childhood lead poisoning that in the United States is often downplayed. She writes for WASAwatch, a blog she founded to keep the public abreast of developments in the unfolding conflict about Washington, DC's unprecedented 2001-2004 lead-at-the-tap crisis and its aftermath.

CHARLES LEVENSTEIN PhD, MSc, is an economist and policy analyst. He is Professor Emeritus in the Department of Work Environment, retiring from teaching in 2003. He is adjunct professor of occupational health at Tufts University School of Medicine and one of the leading researchers concerned with social factors in occupational and environmental health. For several years he was co-director of the Organized Labor and Tobacco Control Consortium, funded by the American Legacy Foundation at Dana Farber Cancer Institute. He subsequently became a consultant to Dr. Edith Balbach's NCI-funded research on tobacco industry relations with trade unions. He has served as member and chair of the environmental health and safety committee of the Massachusetts Teachers Association. He has been engaged in intervention research in immigrant communities and in the economic evaluation of occupational health and safety interventions. Until recently, Dr Levenstein chaired the advisory committee for United Steel Workers federally funded health and safety projects; he continues to chair the advisory board of The New England Consortium, an NIEHS-funded collaboration of health and safety advocacy groups, trade unions and academics. In his most recent edited book, he explores industrial relations systems analysis as an approach to understanding social factors in occupational and environmental health. In his 2002 book (with Greg deLaurier and Mary Lee Dunn), *The Cotton Dust Papers* (2002), he examines the 50-year struggle for recognition of byssinosis ("brown lung") in the United States. Dr. Levenstein served on the IOM/NAS Committee on Health and Safety Needs of Older Workers. He is Editor Emeritus of *New Solutions*, a quarterly peer-reviewed journal of occupational and environmental health policy and is co-editor of the Baywood series on Work, Health and Environment. Prof. Levenstein is a recipient of the American Public Health Association's award for lifetime contribution to occupational health.

BRIAN MAYER, PhD, is an assistant professor of sociology at the University of Arizona. His research interests include environmental sociology, disaster resilience and recovery, medical sociology, and collective behavior and social movements.

RACHEL MORELLO-FROSCH, PhD, is a professor in the Department of Environmental science, Policy and Management and teh School of Public Health at the University of California, Berkeley. Her research integrates environmental health science with social epidemiologic methods to assess potential synergistic effects of social and environmental factors in environmental health disparities. In collaboration with scientific and community colleagues, she has developed scientifically valid and transparent tools for assessing the cumulative impacts of chemical and nonchemical stressors to advance environmental justice goals in regulation and policy. She is assessing the application of these methods for implementation of climate change policies in California.

JOAN N. PARKER was the Director of Safety under Massachusetts Attorneys Generals Scott Harshbarger and Thomas Reilly. In that capacity she was responsible for enforcing the state's laws governing workplace health and safety and child labor. Previously, she investigated workplace health and safety conditions as an industrial hygiene engineer for the Massachusetts Division of Occupational Hygiene. She received a master's degree in industrial health and engineering from the Harvard School of Public Health and was certified as an industrial hygienist by the American Board of Industrial Hygiene.

JEROME PAULSON, MD, is Associate Professor of pediatrics at the George Washington University School of Medicine & Health Sciences and Associate Professor of Prevention and Community Health and Research and of Environmental and Occupational Health at the university's School of Public Health and Health Services. He is the Medical Director for National & Global Affairs of the Child Health Advocacy Institute at the Children's National Medical Center. Dr. Paulson is a co-director of the Mid-Atlantic Center for Children's Health and the Environment. He serves on the American Academy of Pediatrics' Committee on Environmental Health and the Children's Health Protection Advisory Committee for the U.S. Environmental Protection Agency. In October 2004 he was a Dozor Visiting Professor at Ben Gurion University in Beer Sheva, Israel. He was a recipient of a Soros Advocacy Fellowship for Physicians from the Open Society Institute and worked with the Children's Environmental Health Network, and also has served as a special assistant to the director of the National Center on Environmental Health of the Centers for Disease Control and Prevention. He has developed several new courses about children's health and the environment. He has edited several editions of *Pediatric Clinics of North America* on children's environmental health.

EMA RODRIGUES is a postdoctoral fellow in the Environmental and Occupational Medicine and Epidemiology program at Harvard School of Public Health in Boston.

MADELEINE KANGSEN SCAMMELL is an Assistant Professor of Environmental Health at Boston University School of Public Health where she also directs the Community Engagement and Research Translation Cores of the Boston University Superfund Research Program. Her work includes developing long-term mechanisms to support research relationships between community groups and scientists, responding to community requests for assistance from university scientists, and making science relevant to communities and decision-makers dealing with environmental health hazards. Her research interests include developing new analytic methods to study environmental health and cumulative burden, incorporating qualitative social sciences, measurement theory and data representations via lattice structures. Madeleine serves on the Board of Health in the City of Chelsea and is also a member of the board of directors of the Science & Environmental Health Network.

LAURA SENIER holds a joint appointment in the Department of Community and Environmental Sociology and the Department of Family Medicine at the University of Wisconsin–Madison. Her research interests include the sociology of public health and medicine, community environmental health, and environmental justice.

EILEEN SENN is an industrial hygienist who has performed occupational health work for government and unions in New Jersey and Pennsylvania for 38 years. She wrote the seminal article, "Playing Industrial Hygiene to Win," published in *New Solutions* in spring 1991. A spring 2003 update is online at www.nycosh.org/reference_library/Senn.html. She is currently a consultant with the New Jersey Work Environment Council, assisting the New Jersey Education Association with school health and safety issues, and she previously worked for the New Jersey Department of Health and Senior Services in occupational health surveillance for 16 years. Earlier, she was an OSHA inspector in Philadelphia for eight years and worked for the United Auto Workers and the International Brotherhood of Boilermakers providing technical assistance and conducting worker education. Her undergraduate degree is in chemistry from Duquesne University and her master's degree is in industrial hygiene from Temple University.

ANDREA KIDD TAYLOR, DrPH, MSPH, is an assistant professor at Morgan State University's School of Community Health and Policy, and an associate faculty member at the Johns Hopkins University Bloomberg School of Public Health. She has more than 20 years of experience in occupational and environmental health and safety. She served a five-year term as a presidential appointee (Clinton) on the U.S. Chemical Safety and Hazard Investigation Board in Washington, DC (a board patterned after the National Transportation Safety Board to investigate chemical accidents at fixed facilities); and she worked earlier as an industrial hygienist and occupational health policy consultant for the International Union, United Automobile, Aerospace, and Agricultural Implement Workers of America (UAW) in Detroit. She is currently an executive board member of the American Public Health Association and she is a member of the Beyond Pesticides National Advisory Board.

SIMONI TRIANTAFYLLIDOU, MS, is a PhD candidate in Civil Engineering at Virginia Tech. She has more than three years of research experience on the corrosion of drinking water plumbing, as it affects drinking water quality and public health. She has authored and co-authored several publications on various scientific aspects of this problem, most recently in the peer-reviewed journal *Environmental Science and Technology*, regarding the association between lead in water and lead in blood for Washington, DC children in 2001-2004. In 2007, she was awarded the Montgomery-Watson-Harza Consulting Engineers/Association of Environmental Engineering and Science Professors (AEESP) First Place Master's Thesis Award, as well as the American Water Works Association (AWWA) First Place Master's Thesis Academic Achievement Award.

DOROTHY WIGMORE has worked as a health and safety specialist for nearly 30 years in Canada, the United States, and Mozambique. These days, the former journalist and office worker writes, researches, and trains on a variety of health and safety topics, including ergonomics, workplace stressors, green jobs, and integrating occupational and environmental health. Based in Winnipeg, Manitoba, she uses participatory methods for her work, as well as for planning and evaluation activities. Her interest in school-based hazards comes from recent work doing an environmental scan about toxic use reduction activities in Canada and preparing stress and other workshops for the American Federation of Teachers.

JEAN ZOTTER is the Director of the Asthma Prevention and Control Program at the Massachusetts Department of Public Health.

Index